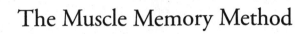

The Muscle Memory Method

The Muscle Memory Method™

*Easy, All-Day Fitness for a
Strong, Firm, Younger Body*

Marjorie Jaffe

with Jo Sgammato

Photographs by George Kerrigan
Illustrations by Roman Szolkowski

M. Evans and Company, Inc.
New York

M. Evans and Company, Inc.

216 East 49th Street

New York, New York 10017

Library of Congress Cataloging-in-Publication Data

Jaffe, Marjorie.

    The muscle memory method : easy, all-day fitness for a strong, firm, younger body / Marjorie Jaffe with Jo Sgammato.

        p.   cm.

    Includes index.

    ISBN 0-87131-819-9

    1. Physical fitness for women. I. Sgammato, Jo. II. Title.

GV482.J34   1997

613.7'045—dc21   96-53168

                                                   CIP

Book design by Annemarie Redmond

Manufactured in the United States of America

9 8 7 6 5 4 3 2 1

DEDICATION

For Mom and Dad, Rena and Sidney
With Love and 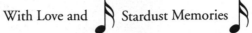 Stardust Memories

"Cogito ergo sum."

I think, therefore I am.

—Descartes

Contents

Doctor's Orders:
Exercise with Marjorie Jaffe

Every time I see Marjorie Jaffe, I stand up straighter.

Why is that?

Since I met Marjorie more than ten years ago, I have been using her Muscle Memory Method for myself and for my patients.

I have been to Marjorie's classes, worked with her privately, and attended her spas in the Catskill Mountains and Jamaica. She practices what she preaches, and she preaches really well.

Marjorie promotes concentrated, focused exercising. She believes that if you exercise correctly, the time you spend goes to much more efficient use. She also believes that posture, alignment, strong muscles, and flexibility keep you young. She keeps people free of neck and back pain.

If you follow Marjorie's program you are much less likely to injure yourself because you have "kinesthetic awareness" and "muscle memory."

As an internist in private practice on the upper west side of Manhattan, I have many patients who are intense, striving, and hardworking. I tell them that as their doctor, it is my job to "worry" about their health. To enormously improve their chances for health, their job is to have regular physical checkups and take whatever tests are recommended, even when they insist they don't need them.

Many of my patients are physically "fit." They belong to gyms, go to step classes, take yoga, and train for marathons. Still, many of these women and men have poor posture and chronic neck, shoulder, and back pain. I'm likely to refer a person with one of these problems to Marjorie.

It's inevitable that we grow older. But if we are vital, flexible, fit, and toned, we don't have to feel or look older. I want to be straight, strong, and elegant as long as I'm here. Subscribing to Marjorie Jaffe's philosophy by reading her book (and, if you're really lucky, meeting her in person) will give you a healthy, supple body.

—Sharon Lewin, M.D.
New York, New York

Part One

CHAPTER ONE
Your Intelligent Key to Fitness

Love Your Muscles

A rewarding relationship with your body will keep you vital, attractive, strong, flexible, and sexual. Intelligent exercise is the key to using your natural strength and grace.

This innovative program is easy, comfortable, and effective. All you need to do is open your mind to accept one concept: If you tell your muscles what to do, they will follow and remember.

Only you can send yourself the message to build a beautiful and healthy body. In this book, I will give you new information and lots of inspiration to achieve a life-long, habit-forming, enjoyable exercise commitment. I will help you feel more relaxed about the exercise process by teaching you a specific program that works. Whatever your prior exercise experience, you can gain lasting fitness through a completely different way of thinking about your muscles and your body.

Hundreds of students who have come to my studio over the past twenty-five years have learned that this is the most satisfying approach to exercise. Many of them comment that the Muscle Memory Method feels like magic. "It's so easy," they say, "but it works."

The magic comes from tapping into the intelligence that exists not only in your brain but in your muscles. This method teaches you to use that intelligence for the only fitness program you'll ever need. You will get greater results with fewer repetitions. Your joints will be flexible. Your bones will stay strong and may even get stronger. Your weight will be easier to manage. You will learn to love your muscles when you see what you get in return for your efforts. With this new approach, you'll find you like the feeling of getting that physical edge.

Sound too good to be true? Well, give me a few minutes to introduce and explain what I call "The Muscle Memory Method," the revolutionary technique that takes a fifteen-minute workout and makes it work for you all day. You'll see that a little extra *mental* stimulation helps you appreciate the pleasure of physical movement.

Your Muscles Possess Intelligence

You've already trained your mind to assimilate new ideas. This is another new one: Your muscles have an intelligence quotient all their own.

Over the years, I have devised hundreds of exercises designed to resist the downward pull of gravity and reverse the signs of aging. These are gentle, intelligent, and effective movements that lengthen your neck; strengthen your chest, upper back, and shoulders; prevent that round-shouldered look; firm your upper arms; slim your waist and hips; and tone your legs and thighs.

To create a beautiful meal, you have to know how to cook. To speak a language fluently, you need to know the words and the grammar. And to use your body intelligently, you have to understand the language of movement as it describes your body's parts and how they all work together.

When I teach, my students learn the names of the muscles, how each muscle works and how to get the most out of each movement. They locate and touch the origin and insertion of each muscle, which I'll show you how to do, too. The secret to effective exercise is not in endless repetitions but in the proper form, conscious intensity, and enjoyment that make exercise a permanent habit. Knowing what you're doing, why and how it benefits you, keeps you involved and motivated.

I call my studio program "Back in Shape" for two reasons. First, it can get anyone, no matter how out of shape, back into the best condition possible. But, more importantly, by concentrating on aligning the back—your spine—into shape, your entire body—from head to toe—is engaged in a process of identifying, feeling, and correctly using all of its muscles.

With this workout, you'll get to know your body from the inside out. You won't feel intimidated. Instead, you'll develop the tools to direct your own fitness and your efforts will be validated by how you look and feel. Integrating your five senses makes this workout a full-bodied, highly engaging experience. Your motivation stays high when you connect your mental and physical processes.

What is "Muscle Memory?"

Muscle Memory occurs in your body when your mind learns a new concept and transmits it to your muscles. Your muscle intelligence assimilates and remembers what the brain communicated to create new muscle habits.

Dancers, athletes, and other performing artists have been using Muscle Memory for many years. Their bodies remember the dance steps or the technique of catching a football long after that last performance or game. When a dancer is sick and can't dance in an important rehearsal, she can watch the rehearsal and then perform the movements flawlessly. When a wide receiver is tired near the end of a game, he uses Muscle Memory to maintain his level of play.

You have Muscle Memory and use it unconsciously all the time. The body remembers how to stand up; it remembers how to ride a bike. For a few days after you rearrange the furniture, your body goes to where the couch used to be. When you move the silverware to a different drawer, you go to the original drawer until the new positions set in and your muscles adjust.

For years, I have taught my students to use the mind–body connection to enhance their fitness efforts. Now I have formalized this approach into the total Muscle Memory Method exercise program for them—and for you.

How Does It Work?

The Muscle Memory Method takes place in two stages: first, practice an exercise that trains the muscle correctly and, second, reinforce that correct muscle usage throughout your day. When you train your muscles to take over, exercise becomes easier. The awareness of the mental–physical connection helps you recruit more muscle fibers.

For example, you use your quadriceps, the big muscle on the front of your thigh, when walking up stairs. Until now you may have done that unconsciously. Now, with the Muscle Memory Method, the simple act of walking up the stairs adds to your fitness level.

Using Muscle Memory, you will be able to align your body to defy gravity and look better than you ever have before. I'll explain how this works in Chapter Two. Students tell me that as soon as they hear even one Muscle Memory tip during exercise instructions, their "alignment buttons" are pressed and every body part moves into the correct position.

Unlike other exercise programs you may have tried and abandoned, my Muscle Memory Method techniques produce lasting results because you learn how to be in control of your own fitness. After mastering Muscle Memory, you'll become smarter about your physical condition, and you'll no longer have to rely on someone telling you how to exercise. You'll become your own personal trainer.

THE CHALLENGE

Whether you hardly ever touch your toes or you work out constantly, time will make changes to your body that you will want to learn to monitor. You want to keep your shoulders and neck straight, tummy pulled in, and hips and thighs lean and strong. Exercise is the best way to accomplish this.

If you are sedentary and don't use your body, it's possible to gain one pound of fat and lose one-half pound of lean body mass per year after the age of twenty-five. We can counteract this by exercising and keeping our metabolic rate (the rate at which we burn calories) high.

The force of gravity is forever surrounding and affecting us. If you were holding a pencil and let it go, it would drop to the floor immediately. Gravity affects our bodies in the same way. Sitting all day increases the gravitational pull on all of our muscles. When we stand, we are subject to 100 percent gravity. Lying down, we don't have to fight gravity. But when we sit, we lower our center of gravity and compact our bodies. Then we face the equivalent of 150 percent of normal gravitational pull on all parts of our bodies.

A muscle that's toned is firm. If your muscles weaken and lose tone, they become soft. That round-shouldered look is one result of softer muscles. Your body can become wider, too, which you notice when your clothes become harder to button.

But a weaker, fatter body is *not* inevitable as you age. Muscles weaken when you use them infrequently or incorrectly. By using the Muscle Memory Method to be muscle-specific in your workout, you'll sharpen your muscle intelligence. This will keep your shoulders straighter, your belly flatter, and your hips narrower. Muscles are the motors that create motion. When the abdominal muscles contract and pull in during exercise, they move the hips and ribs closer together to prevent that "middle-age spread."

At each age, we have an opportunity to ensure a healthier future. What you do in your twenties, thirties, and forties will affect you later on so the best way to have a healthy old age is to have a healthy middle age. It's a good time to increase your awareness of your body's needs. You can maintain bone strength and create new bone cells with the Muscle Memory Method program. Adding aerobic exercise in it's simplest form—walking—and eating a nutritious diet will help you keep a high ratio of muscle cells to fat cells.

Our estrogen levels decrease when we enter menopause, and the testosterone that is a natural part of our body chemistry can play a greater role. That's why some women who have never had fat on their bellies before begin to mimic the male pattern of a wider belly. This exercise program teaches you how to draw in the pelvic muscles as a permanent habit and combat that spread, and how to use your abdominal and back muscles to keep the rib cage lifted.

You can lessen the severity of many of the diseases generally associated with aging. For example, osteoporosis has become a major problem for many women over fifty. This condition sets in when bone loses its mineral mass and progressively becomes porous and brittle. Bones support the structure of your entire body. Weaker bones cannot withstand the stresses of normal living and are more likely to fracture.

This book will help you fight osteoporosis. You'll learn how to keep your bones in a straight line, which will make them less vulnerable to wearing out. These exercises strengthen and stretch the muscles surrounding each joint, keeping it stable. Deep breathing to relax, aerobic conditioning, healthful nutrition, and weight management also fight osteoporosis in a profoundly successful way.

Sensual and Sexy Forever? Yes!

As women today, we are able to view mid-life and menopause not as the end of our womanhood but as the beginning of a whole new phase of life. It can be a time of accomplishment and spirituality, confidence and vigor, sensual experiences, and sexual pleasure. What a great reason to exercise to keep *all* your muscles primed for action! Chapter Seven, Mindsets and Exercises for Sensuality and Sexuality, offers information to increase your sensuality and keep you comfortable with your sexuality. I'll teach you exercises specifically designed to increase your mobility and pleasure.

Small Investment, Big Return

Your body works like a bank account. You have to keep making deposits if you want to stay ahead of the withdrawals. Exercise is a "deposit," an investment in yourself. By doing the Daily Ten Muscle Memory Method Workout (almost) every day, you will see a tremendous return on your investment.

Think of my program as the key to your strong, attractive body. And think of that body as the vessel in which you live the best, most active, and rewarding life you can through your thirties, forties, fifties, sixties, and well beyond.

Recent news reports confirm that we are living a lot longer than we used to. Images of how we'll look and feel at different ages abound in our information-rich and goal-oriented society. I'd like to suggest a different viewpoint. Your personal experience of every decade of life will have much more to do with your own perspective, how you feel physically, and how you present yourself to the world. Exercising now—whether to maintain your fitness or to establish it for the first time—will prepare you to be your best throughout your life.

One of the wonderful things about learning to nurture your health and take more time to do things for yourself is that you see results almost instantly. It's also terrific to know you're storing up some benefits for the future. Decreases in muscle tone, cardiovascular fitness, and bone strength can begin to happen long before we see any outward evidence. Rather than waiting until a medical test shows a decrease in function, embrace the exercise prescription. It's the natural way to prevent your health from declining.

It's never too late—or too early—to make big changes in your health and fitness patterns. I know that a lot of people don't exercise. I know many who do it only because they feel they have to. I've heard of women who began to exercise, injured themselves, and gave it up forever within the first few weeks. If you were to fall off a horse the first time you rode and did not have good instruction on how to prevent another fall, you probably would never mount a horse again. It's the same with exercise, especially if you didn't even like it to begin with.

My goal is to show you how to enjoy and appreciate your workout by making it as simple and effective as possible. You don't need to join a gym, purchase expensive equipment, or go jogging in the rain. All you need is a thick blanket or mat on the floor and your innate brain and muscle intelligence.

Ten Exercises in Only Fifteen Minutes a Day

I know that one of our most precious commodities is time. And we all want to get the most for our exercise time. That's why I've selected the ten most effective exercises to achieve the results you want in only fifteen minutes a day. (I've heard some working mothers and people in high-pressure careers say they're so busy they hardly ever have fifteen minutes all at once. See "Maximizing Your Results" in Chapter Three for help.)

For the Daily Ten, I've chosen the exercises that most effectively work specific parts of your body while toning the entire body at the same time. I've put them in order so that one movement leads gracefully into the next. In words and pictures, I'll give you clear and complete instructions to each of the ten exercises so that you understand how to do them correctly, using your brain and muscle intelligence to reinforce Muscle Memory.

Because every contraction requires an opposite and equal relaxation, I've devised three Recovery Stretches to do between some of the exercises. It adds up to a program that is easy and works in harmony with your body.

In the beginning, your task will be to make each exercise fit *your* body. As you become more familiar with the workout, you'll develop a routine that becomes second nature to you. You'll like how you look and feel, and the "should I or shouldn't I" choice is eliminated.

Ever dream about an exercise program that works when you're sitting still? Well, this is it and here's why.

MUSCLE MEMORY

As you do each of the exercises, you will "program" your muscles with the "memory" of proper shape and usage. For each exercise, your mind will ask and your body will answer relevant questions from the Muscle Memory Quiz that train your own Muscle Memory Voice. The Muscle Memory Voice is a central component of the program because you call on it throughout your day to check that particular muscles are maintaining correct form.

In Chapter Two, you'll learn more about using muscle intelligence. Your mind and your body take the memory of how your muscles looked and felt during the workout with you in all of your daily activities.

While you're standing on line in a store, sitting at your desk, lounging on the couch watching television, driving in your car, or going about your errands and chores, you call on your Muscle Memory to continuously align your body and strengthen your muscles. Say you're at a party or an important business meeting. How wonderful to have the muscle intelligence to stand tall, pull in that belly, straighten those shoulders, and look strong and confident.

You'll look better because you are constantly shaping and contouring your body. You'll feel terrific as you use Muscle Memory to pull your shoulders back, tighten your stomach, draw your hips closer together and elongate your thigh muscles. It's instant! You are using your muscles as anti-gravitational devices.

With the Muscle Memory Method, you can look better even on days when you're under the weather or during those inevitable times when you put on a few extra pounds. Muscle Memory can make you *look* great even when you don't *feel* great.

How will you know when the Muscle Memory program is working for you? Look in the mirror and compare your posture with the picture of the skeleton on page 24. Use the One-Minute Muscle Memory Boost in Chapter Three several times a day to check that your entire body is in alignment.

Complements to the "Muscle Memory" Workout

My students enjoy the Stretch and Joint Looseners in their classes because stretching apart our bodies always feels terrific. Stretching is a must to maintain a healthy spine and supple joints. We'll stretch the usual spots like your back, neck, and shoulders but I'll also show you how to rotate all your joints and open up your chest, ribs, and hips. The Three-Minute Breathing Relaxation can be done anytime, anywhere, and is incredibly effective in combating stress. Breathing deeply can help maintain your upright posture. You'll find these complements in Chapter Four.

Aerobic and Weight-Training Components

Aerobic exercise is vital. If you're tired of focusing on the details of carbohydrate, protein, and fat percentages in your diet, why not try burning *more* calories rather than eating fewer? There is no scientific proof that as we age we must gain weight. It's true that our metabolism decreases each year but it is truer still that exercise raises our metabolism. All of us have a "set" weight at which our bodies are comfortable. This is why it takes a few days to gain weight if we're overeating and a few days to begin showing a weight loss.

I'd like you to include an easy-to-fit-in aerobic walk using the Intelligent Walking Program in Chapter Six. Bringing Muscle Memory to your walk and applying target heart rate in a personalized way will make your walk extra-effective in managing your weight and keeping your heart healthy. Walking also contributes to bone strength.

Strength training is valuable three times a week for additional bone density and muscle shaping. Chapter Five outlines special arm, wrist, and foot exercises you can do with or without weights. Studies have shown that regular weight-bearing exercises not only retard bone loss but can actually increase bone mass. Strength-training exercises increase your muscle strength and power and enhance the muscle shape and contour.

Built-In Willpower

You're always hearing that you need willpower to maintain a consistent exercise routine. My experience is that information and understanding make all the difference. The motivation is clear: You want to look and feel better, increase energy and stamina, and try to prevent illnesses.

Willpower is a renewable resource with the Muscle Memory approach because throughout the workout and throughout the day as you continue to shape and use your muscles properly, you see and feel results all the time. Seeing your body look leaner and feeling your clothes fit more comfortably are satisfactions that translate into the willpower to keep you going.

Exercise to Live

Exercise is not an end in itself. It's the road to the active, vibrant life you want to keep living.

I don't teach aerobics in my studio because people don't need to pay me to move around. There's a world of water to swim in, hillsides to hike, skating ponds, roller rinks, and tennis games to enjoy. There are treadmills, stationery bikes, and ski machines to use to move your body.

People come to me for the exercises that make their muscles stronger and more flexible so that they can improve performance and achieve enjoyment in their sports, outdoor activities, and every other aspect of their lives. When your muscles are toned, you have the confidence to go out and use them for fun. Strong hips and legs make your hike easier. Your golf swing improves noticeably when your upper arms have strength and your joints are flexible. When your chest and back muscles are strong, your tennis serve is strong, too. The Muscle Memory Method trains your muscles to be ready for action. "Muscle readiness" increases your playing ability.

Fitness is the sum total of all your ways of living. Getting older is easier if you're armed with the tools to help you take on new challenges. Rollerblading at fifty? Why not? I'll get you in shape to do it.

Start for Vanity, Continue for Sanity

Spending time and money taking care of yourself—whether it's on your hair, nails, skin, or body—might seem to some people like vanity. Vanity in this case is not one of the seven deadly sins. Rather, it can be a powerful motivator. And even though you might start exercising out of vanity, exercise lifts your spirit so much that you want to recapture that great feeling.

When you connect your physical training to your spiritual well-being, you can become more centered and focused. You'll find help and a special meditation for this in Chapter Four. Tiredness from physical exhaustion doesn't feel like fatigue; it feels like exhilaration. Your body may be tired but your mind is energetic.

The Muscle Memory Method requires a dialogue between your brain and your muscles to function in harmony and balance. This integration of the mind and body can make you feel powerful. The exercises heighten the ability of your nerve cells to respond to stimuli. This makes you more self-aware and then more aware of everything around you.

Many of my students rely on my classes to keep their heads in shape as much as their backs and bodies. Exercise improves your mood profoundly. It decreases stress hormones and increases natural mood-lifting chemicals. Exercise is much better than overeating when you need to relax and overcome stress.

Every Age Can Be Fabulous!

I don't believe in the fantasy that you can look twenty-nine your whole life. Muscles cannot keep *all* of their firmness forever. But I know—and I've seen it proven time and again in my studio—that intelligent exercise will help you look attractive and firm, fit into your clothes well, and keep you doing the activities you enjoy. It's time now to develop the sort of relationship with your muscles that you enjoy with your closest friends.

Even though you may never have thought of yourself as a "physical" person, your body can look better now than ever before.

So, let's get started!

CHAPTER TWO
Laying the Foundation for Muscle Memory

If you could do something quickly and easily every day to look and feel better, wouldn't you? Your body seeks comfort and can be very responsive to intelligent exercise instructions. I'm going to help you learn about your muscles in a new way. Your Daily Ten Workout uses the major muscle groups correctly, so they remember proper form when you walk, sit, and stand.

I've paid attention to people's intelligence during the last twenty-five years of teaching exercise. When I teach students to hear their own voices and learn to give themselves instructions while exercising, they're able to recall instant alignment and muscle tone on their own. Develop your own Muscle Memory Voice and you'll be able to do the same.

Alignment is stacking your bones in a straight line, beginning with your feet up through your head, and holding that line straight with your muscles. In years past, this is what was called "good posture." It is the basis for what we now call Muscle Memory.

Students embrace this method enthusiastically when I tell them it's 70 percent intellectual and 30 percent physical—once your mind understands it, your body responds. Always tight for time, they enjoy the appearance and extra energy they instantly get with this program. In Chapter Three, as you learn the exercises, I'll teach you the questions from the Muscle Memory Quiz to ask yourself about specific parts of your body. Then I'll show you how to get the right answers.

Muscle Memory:
- *You teach your muscles what to do during exercise and they remember.*
- *Your mind conveys the correct anatomical information and sends the message of healthy habits into the muscles.*
- *You keep in mind where the muscles are and what they do, so they'll always work for you.*
- *You recognize and utilize the intelligence quotient of your muscle fibers.*

Your body can do what your mind sets it to.

HOW TO TRAIN MUSCLE MEMORY

At the beginning, you may find the following concepts complicated and wonder how you'll remember everything. Muscle Memory is a new language. Once you learn it, the program

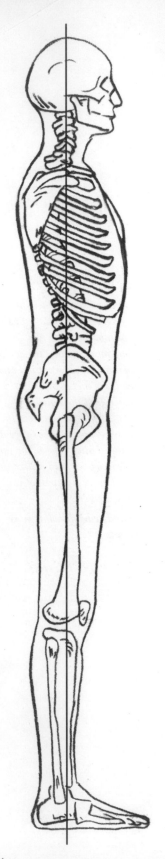

becomes simple. This has worked countless times before and will become a new habit for you. You're learning to direct your body back to its natural grace.

There are over 400 skeletal muscles in your body that you control. Automatic, split-second communication takes place constantly between your eye, your brain, and your muscles. *Your mind sends messages to your body.* The muscles have the intelligence to respond by taking the shape and form that the mind directs.

The instructions for each of the Daily Ten include a sidebar showing where each muscle begins (the *origin*) and where it ends (the *insertion*). You'll feel the work in the middle (the *belly*) of the muscle.

Your body is a continuous chain of muscles. If you stretch your neck, you feel it down at your tail. Making just one movement causes a chain reaction that gets the whole body moving. This chain reaction gives you additional strength and enhances the Muscle Memory Method. Although each of the ten exercises targets a primary muscle, the entire body is involved whenever one muscle works.

The following directions apply not only to all the exercises in this book, they are meant to become part of your mindset. Your goal is to be able to recruit muscle fibers automatically. This comes from that ongoing communication between your brain cells and your muscle cells. Once you feel the muscles that control alignment and become familiar with the feeling, new muscle habits will take hold and you'll need to think less about the process. Muscle Memory will take care of any corrections.

Synchronize your mental and physical processes to train the *nerve-to-muscle* impulse we call Muscle Memory. Muscles are cellular motors that move all parts of your body. When you exercise using Muscle Memory, you shape the muscle into its proper form. When you're standing or sitting or walking, your muscles remember to perform because they've been there before.

Learn how to communicate directions to your body to stand tall with your ribs lifted out of your hips, with your belly in and your neck and shoulders relaxed for instant Muscle Memory.

Your body is a brilliant machine meant to move. Learn to be aware of each movement and which muscles produce it. Did you know that each muscle is part of a pair that always work together? When a muscle is weak, its "partner" has to work twice as hard in an unnatural way that often produces tension and/or pain. Your best defense against pain and injury is a well-conditioned body. Increased stamina contributes to your performance potential. Conditioned muscles look shaped and firm while de-conditioned ones look soft and flabby. This program gives you better performance and therapeutic, as well as aesthetic, benefits.

THE ALIGNMENT CHECK-UP

Stand sideways to a mirror—full-length, if possible—and match your alignment to the illustration of the skeleton. Your eyes send visual messages to your brain, which then directs your muscles to work.

There are five alignment checkpoints—at the ankles, knees, hips, shoulders and ears—to see if you're standing up straight. Check that each part is in a straight line with the others. Begin by placing your weight toward the balls of your feet and then balance the weight of your body over the arches. Notice how your body is balanced in an even front and back half.

When you lie down, you'll find it easier to practice aligning yourself. The downward gravitational pull is eliminated so you don't need to expend energy to hold yourself up. Strengthen the specific alignment muscles while lying down and, using Muscle Memory, achieve alignment while standing up.

Body Planes

A body has three basic planes relating to dimensions in space, which are at right angles to each other. Each divides the body in equal halves. They are:

1. Sagittal Plane—divides into right and left halves
2. Coronal Plane—divides into front and back halves
3. Transverse Plane—divides into upper and lower halves

Follow the illustration and divide your body into the three planes. The point at which they intersect is the *center of gravity*, right behind your navel. Relating your body awareness to this point at all times—during exercise and during the rest of your day—will help you feel centered and focused. Your body will

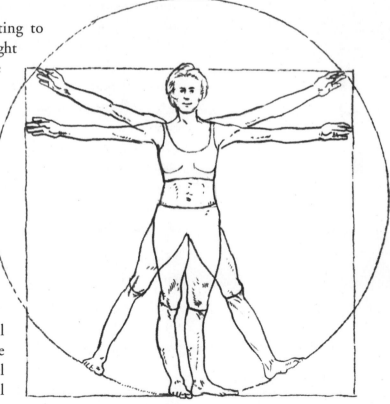

look balanced. You'll have more energy because you're using the maximum amount of muscles correctly. You won't strain yourself by making one muscle do more work than it's meant to in compensating for the weaker ones.

Body Segment Balance

Remember that the body is designed on the basis of a right and left half, a front and back half, and an upper and lower half. If you were to draw a body on graph paper, it would line up in a straight line and you'd be able to separate each body segment into quarters.

Think of a vertical line dropping through the center of each body segment from your head to your feet. Visualize this concept. Put your hands on your head and divide it into a front and back half and a left and right half. As the two planes intersect each other, your head has four equal sections. Do this with each segment of your body: your chest and upper back, the front and back of your ribcage, the front and back of your pelvis, the front and back of your knees, and the front and back of your feet.

The movement on one half will automatically move the other half. For example, when the ribs pull down in front, the ribs in back automatically tilt up. Or if you were to lift the ribs in the back, the front would automatically tilt down. The correct anatomical position for the rib cage is to be pointed down in the front and lifted in the back. Look at the picture of the skeleton and you'll see what I mean.

This follows through for all the segments in the body. When the pubic bone tilts up, the tailbone tilts down. Put your hands on your hips. Feel the front and back points and draw a horizontal line between them.

This specific anatomical information is the underpinning of each of the Daily Ten. Much of it happens unconsciously whenever you work a muscle. However, when you're conscious of what's happening in your exercise, you can apply this knowledge and use it all the time. Check it by answering your Muscle Memory Quiz.

Muscle Balance

All muscles produce movement the same way: They pull in and contract. The contraction pulls on the tendons (at the end of each muscle) which, in turn, move your bones. Muscles work in pairs. One cannot work alone. For every muscle that contracts, there's an opposing muscle that relaxes. Contracting is pulling in, relaxing is releasing. For example, when your biceps contracts to bend your arm, the triceps on the underarm relaxes.

Hip and knee problems are prevalent today because of muscle imbalance. Striving for muscle balance now can help prevent these problems later on.

Learn to be aware of which muscles produce each movement. The fact that two muscles work at the same time produces a double benefit each time you exercise because it makes more muscle cells work. You'll see what I mean in each of the ten exercises.

Body Spaces

We all admire a dancer's body. One quality that makes it so attractive is the swan-like neck. Make this a part of your look by increasing the space between your ear and shoulders and strengthening the muscles that maintain it. The space between your ribs and hips that defines your waistline also contributes to that long, lean look. Maintaining these two spaces keeps your muscles from getting crunched up and irritating the nerves. Look good and prevent pain at the same time!

The muscle on the back of the arm (triceps) originates underneath the shoulder blade and inserts at the elbow. Pulling the arm up lifts the rib cage. Because the thigh bone fits into the hip bone, pulling the leg down also pulls down the hip. Together these motions increase the space between the ribs and the hips.

Use your hands to measure the linear distances on your body. Put your thumb on your shoulder and third finger on your ear to lengthen the space between them. Place your thumb in the belly button and third finger on your pubic bone to check that the abdominal muscles are pulled in and tight. With your thumb on your breast bone and pinkie in your belly button, tighten the rectus abdominis muscle that runs up and down the front of your belly. Then feel your concave belly from breast bone to pubic bone.

Muscle Fibers

Muscle fibers are arranged in a specific spatial design. That's why some abdominal exercises move straight up and down and others twist diagonally to follow the pattern of the fibers. Keep this in mind throughout the exercises so you can visualize the motion and be sure to move in a compatible direction. When you exercise correctly—with your muscles and not against them—you achieve greater benefits, reduce soreness, and sustain your interest and ability.

Keeping the Body Narrow

Think of wrapping in your muscles. Visualize the red and blue stripes wrapping around an old-fashioned barber's pole and match that feeling by integrating and combining the front and the back of your body. Apply that vision to the lower abdominal muscles that pull the hips in tight to stay slim and narrow. You'll understand this better when you do the abdominal exercises in the Daily Ten.

Gravity's Effects—And Effectiveness

In our exercises, we hold ourselves up against the downward pull of gravity. This adds intensity to each movement, making it more effective. We acknowledge gravity and lean into it for a greater stretch. The gravity that pulls us down also works for us by making our bones stronger—and by keeping us from floating away. When a muscle pulls on a bone, the bone increases in density.

"Good" Versus "Bad" Tension

Muscle tension is good when you're doing it on purpose. Contracting, pulling in, shortening, and tensing are the synonymous verbs for working a muscle. A muscle gets stronger as you tense it. Be aware, however, that every contraction needs the same amount of relaxation time so the muscle doesn't weaken. Be careful not to tense your muscles unconsciously. When your shoulders are lifted too close to your ears, learn to drop them. Acknowledge neck tension in your life, when you're shortening, hunching, and bunching those important neck muscles. Think of "tension" as holding a muscle and "relaxation" as letting go.

There are strategies you can employ as you're learning the Muscle Memory Method to make it work faster. For instance, hold a ruler or a piece of paper behind your head and check that the head is in the same line as your upper back. Place your hand in front of your chest to check that your chest is in front of your stomach. These are just two of the many strategies you'll find in the answers to the Muscle Memory Quiz.

At every moment, be mindful. Whether absorbed in a Picasso painting or waiting for an appointment, take a moment to fix your body with Muscle Memory. Keep copies of the Muscle Memory Quiz handy and check it several times a day. After all, you don't want to *undo* the muscle toning you attained when you exercised. The less time you spend slumped and hunched, the less damage you have to undo when you're exercising. The less you have to undo during your workout, the more you will accomplish.

Fit Fitness into Every Day

Everything you do contributes to your fitness level. Put as much physical activity as you can into your daily life. Even a ten-minute walk three times a day will make a difference. Muscles can shut down simply from disuse. We are in many sedentary positions each day. Stand up and walk around whenever you can.

I know that as you evolve through this program, you will become a more physical person. The fitter you are, the easier it is to stay in shape. The better you feel as a result of physical activity, the more motivated you'll be to stay with it.

Much as I want you to add fitness to your life, I also want to caution you not to abandon your other interests. We have a limited amount of leisure time and want to satisfy all of our curiosities. Sometimes people who become interested in fitness for the first time become addicted to it. Soon it becomes a burden and they give it up. Strive for balance. Let fitness be one of many wonderful parts of your life.

Use Your Intelligence

These are new concepts, new ways of looking at exercise. People who have never exercised before—and even many who have—may not be aware that the space between the ear and the shoulder is an issue. But once you realize the profound importance of that simple concept to the whole look, feel, and health of your body, you are ready to learn more.

This book is designed to give you the knowledge to self-direct your body. There are many of you who have put children, families, academic studies, and professional ambition ahead of your own needs. You're proud of your achievements. But now you have the desire to be healthy, to live longer and better.

Here are the tools you may have missed along the way because you were so busy. I want you to use the intelligence you used in other aspects of your life to benefit your health and body. You know how to learn. You've learned more difficult things in your life than exercise.

You know how to integrate intelligent exercise information into your life—especially now that you realize how much it will benefit you.

Part Two

CHAPTER THREE

The Muscle Memory
Method Workout

GETTING STARTED

The Muscle Memory Method is so different from other exercise programs that you really need to take some time to get to know it before getting started. As an experienced exercise teacher, I'm giving you a lot of information in this book. I encourage you to develop your own Muscle Memory Voice.

If in an hour-long class in my studio I use many more than ten exercises to keep students interested, why is it that ten are enough for you? How do only ten exercises work to keep all your muscles fit and toned? They take advantage of the body's three-dimensional aspect, using your front, back, and sides with each exercise. The Daily Ten tone all our basic muscle groups: the upper and lower abdominals...upper, middle, and lower back...neck, chest, and shoulders...front, back, inner, and outer sides of arms and legs.

How does this program deliver such great results? The emphasis is on body alignment and correct form while focusing on flexibility, strength, balance, and endurance. These are very creative exercises. One of my students, who is an artist, said, "Many of the exercises we do work the same muscles differently. It's as if I were sculpting a piece and turned it over to achieve a different look."

Even though I know hundreds of different exercises, I feel comfortable telling you that these ten will keep your muscles in great shape.

Soon, your new habits of keeping the abdominals pulled in and head lifted tall, will replace your old habits automatically. Slumping will feel unnatural to you.

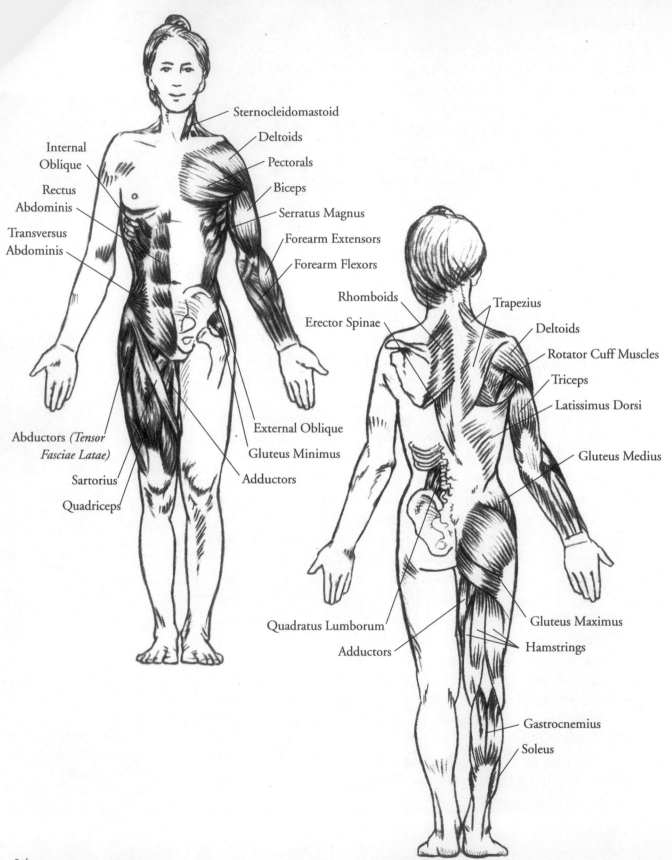

Sternocleidomastoid

Deltoids

Pectorals

Biceps

Serratus Magnus

Forearm Extensors

Forearm Flexors

Internal
Oblique

Rectus
Abdominis

Transversus
Abdominis

Rhomboids

Erector Spinae

Trapezius

Deltoids

Rotator Cuff Muscles

Triceps

Latissimus Dorsi

Gluteus Medius

External Oblique

Gluteus Minimus

Adductors

Abductors *(Tensor
Fasciae Latae)*

Sartorius

Quadriceps

Quadratus Lumborum

Adductors

Gluteus Maximus

Hamstrings

Gastrocnemius

Soleus

Gain Without Pain

Acknowledge the right to feel comfortable as you exercise. The exercise that feels comfortable is the only one to do. If an exercise does not feel right, it may not fit your body well. I'll show you how to solve that.

Some days you might not be in the mood or too busy to do all of the Daily Ten. I've broken it into three Five-Minute Workouts, which you'll find later in this chapter. Choose one.

After you've mastered the Daily Ten, stay with them. You don't have to keep looking for more and harder exercises to do. In fact, over-training can abuse your muscles and joints. But if you're brand new to exercise, start slowly. Your body will soon become knowledgeable and respond appropriately.

Acknowledge Your Preferences

Match your exercise routine to your preferences and you'll enjoy it much more. There's no rule about what time and where you "should" exercise. Do you want your workout time to be scheduled or flexible? Do you feel better exercising alone or with a friend? Wear what makes you feel good—or exercise naked. Think about your preferences. Try working out with music and with silence and see which feels better to you. At times, I like music because it elicits an emotional response that completes the mind-body-spirit connection.

Give yourself permission to take a break from time to time and you'll find that you feel more relaxed about your fitness regime.

PREPARE TO LEARN THE EXERCISES

The Muscle Memory program relies on the involvement of your mind as much as your body. Seventy percent mental knowledge plus 30 percent physical training adds up to 100 percent of Muscle Memory.

One student, a forty-plus attorney, said, "The thought is the mother of all ideas. The mind has to experience an idea several times and then it will accept it."

So here's what I'd like you to do with each exercise before you even move a muscle.

First the Mind, Then the Body

Look at the anatomical drawing and the sidebar to locate and identify the muscles used in the exercise and the origin and insertion of those muscles. Familiarize yourself with the names of the muscles. This helps your muscles remember the exercise value all day. My students tell me they enjoy learning these names and that this method stimulates and enhances their workout (they even use the names in games of Scrabble).

Read the instructions carefully and visualize the motions. Look at the photographs in which I demonstrate the exercise (after all, a picture is still worth a thousand words). Then imagine yourself going through each step.

After you understand the exercise intellectually, do it slowly and refer to the sidebar, "Your Muscle Memory Voice." These are the selected questions from the Muscle Memory Quiz you'll soon learn how to answer.

Using Origin and Insertion

Use your hands now. Locate the origin and insertion of the muscle. As you'll recall from Chapter Two, the origin is the point where the muscle begins and the insertion is the point where it ties into the body. Between those two points is the belly of the muscle, the spot at which you direct your effort to increase the size and number of muscle fibers. Feel that the origin is stable, the insertion is moving, and the muscle fibers are working. Touching ensures you are targeting a specific muscle and not mindlessly using momentum. When the muscle produces a very tiny movement, feel the bone moving so you know something is working.

In some exercises, the origin and insertion principle can be used differently to gain additional benefits. After using the origin to stabilize, pull it in the opposite direction from the insertion. The hamstring muscle functions like a rubber band. Picture pulling a rubber band apart at both ends instead of from one end only. You get maximum stretch in the middle and a longer rubber band. In the Hamstring Strengthener, move the hip away from the insertion at the knee as you work for a greater stretch. We all want long muscles and this is one way to get them.

Applying the origin and insertion principle, you benefit from the positive chain reaction. One mental command initiates a response from the many muscles that work together to create alignment.

Customize Each Movement

Remember to make each exercise fit *your* body. Imagine yourself trying on a new suit and pulling it down here, up there, making it sit correctly over your chest, through the waistline, and around your hips. The same exercise fits each body differently, so nip here, tuck there, and move around until you feel comfortable. That's when you'll know it's right for you.

Look for the movements and positions in each exercise that you can transfer to your daily life. Think about what you're doing during each exercise so you can recall it during the day. When you're aware of using your hamstring during an exercise, you'll use it correctly when you're walking or playing sports, giving you more power and preventing injury to your knee.

Give a final extra squeeze to the muscle at the end of each movement and feel it "set." Squeeze your hand into a fist and copy the sensation that you feel into the target muscle.

Breathing

Breathe in and out in a relaxed way. Inhale deeply as you begin to initiate the exercise mentally. Then exhale forcefully into the belly of the working muscle. Let go in-between and repeat this breathing pattern. We naturally inhale, but sometimes forget to exhale deeply. This is important because we make room for fresh air when we eliminate the used air in our lungs.

Your Muscle Memory Voice

While mastering the physical form of each exercise, pay close attention to your Muscle Memory Voice. This communication between your mind and your muscles is the essential component that keeps your form correct and makes the Daily Ten work. For the first five exercises, there are three questions from the Muscle Memory Quiz to ask yourself. Over the next four exercises, you'll increase the number of questions. Finally, with the last one, the Shoulder Circles, you'll ask all ten of the Muscle Memory Quiz questions. Refer to the answers on pages 68–70 for help in imprinting your Muscle Memory.

By keeping your mind fully present during each exercise, you maintain focus and increase your Muscle Memory. Throughout your day, answer the Muscle Memory Quiz wherever you are, whatever you're doing, and reinforce your answers with the One-Minute Muscle Memory Boost.

Soon, you'll understand fully, maybe for the first time in your life, the fabulous feeling and the long, lean look that come with proper alignment. Results will happen quickly with this program but I encourage you to move away from a "quick fix" mentality. Instead, embrace the pleasures and satisfactions of a long-time, habit-forming exercise commitment.

Success comes at different times. This program is about developing a real working relationship with your body that you can count on.

LEARN how to develop your voice.

USE it as you do your daily workout.

REMEMBER and APPLY it all day.

Your Muscle Memory Voice is what you take with you from the exercise workout. The understanding is what makes it work.

The Muscle Memory Quiz

1. Are there two long spaces in my body: Between my ear and shoulder? Between my ribs and hips?

2. Is the back of my head in the same line as my upper back?

3. Do my shoulders point straight to the ceiling?

4. Do I feel the same strength in my chest and upper back?

5. Am I pulling my ribs in front down and lifting the ribs in back?

6. Is my chest more forward than my belly?

7. Is my pubic bone pulling up and tail bone tilting down?

8. Are my leg muscles balanced so my knee is aligned and not stiff?

9. Are my feet balanced? Is the center of my body directly above my arches?

10. Can I drop a plumb line from the ceiling and have it go down the center of each body segment in a straight line?

The Daily Ten:
The Muscle Memory Method
Workout

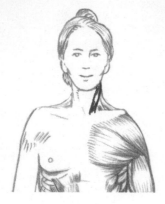

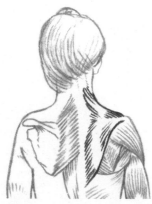

Primary Muscles Used:

Side and Back of Neck

Muscle: Trapezius
Origin: Spine of middle back
Insertion: Shoulder and head

Muscle: Sternocleidomastoid
Origin: Breastbone (sternum)
Insertion: Bone behind ear
(mastoid)

Neck Lengtheners

The anthropologist Margaret Mead said we can tell what's important in a culture by how often it is referred to. How about that classic "pain in the neck?" You need space for the seven vertebrae in your neck. If neck muscles tense and shorten, your neck hunches and the nerves radiating from the vertebrae become irritated and cause pain. Throughout this exercise, be aware of the length of your spine, from your neck all the way down to your tailbone.

Number
Three repetitions, alternating each side.

Position
Lie on your back with knees bent, feet flat on floor. Bend your elbows and place your hands near top of head.

Breathing
Inhale as you lift your head. Exhale as you turn.

Instructions
1. Bring your elbows forward and slide the back of your neck as straight down as possible onto the floor. Engage the trapezius to hold your shoulders back and pull your shoulder blades down.

2. Bend your head down and use your hands to help lift it slightly so the weight of your head is lifted but hair still touches floor. (Figure 1)

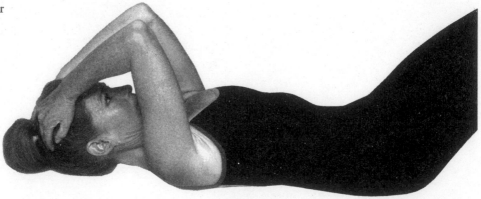

Figure 1

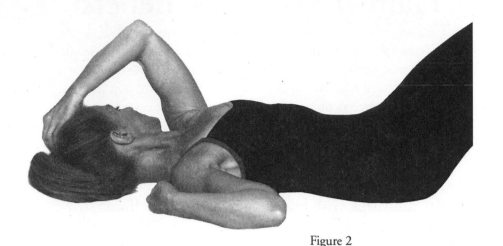

Figure 2

Your Muscle Memory Voice

➤ *Is there a long space between my ear and shoulder? Between my ribs and hips?*
➤ *Do I feel the same strength in my chest and upper back?*
➤ *Is my pubic bone pulling up and tail bone tilting down?*

3. Leading with the left hand, turn and look over your left shoulder, keeping your head in the center of your body. Move your right hand to your right shoulder to press it down. (Figure 2)

4. Return to center. Change hands and repeat on the other side.

5. Drop your head down and wobble it to relax.

A Strong Neck Maintains Grace and Comfort All Day

When tension strikes your neck and gravity impacts there, move your head back and lift it to lengthen and strengthen your neck muscles. Call on your Muscle Memory to increase the space between your ear and shoulder. Use your fingertips and massage your neck muscles deeply. If you can, lie down to eliminate the tension of holding up your head. Instant comfort!

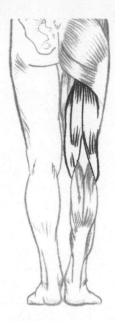

Primary Muscle Used:

Hamstring

Muscle: Hamstring
Origin: Bottom of hip
Insertion: Back of knee

Hamstring Strengtheners

Not wanting to be "hamstrung" (dictionary definition: disabled), we do this exercise for the strength and flexibility we need in every step we take and for most other exercises. Avoid the hamstring injuries that cause many professional athletes to miss performances. Think of how nice it is to stretch to pick up something and reach it easily.

Number
Steps 1–4, five times; step 5, eight times.

Position
Lie on your back with knees bent, feet flat on floor, arms at side.

Breathing
Inhale on the stretch. Exhale as you straighten.

Instructions
1. Stretch your right arm straight over your head. Drop your right leg, point your toes, and lift your leg an inch from floor. Stretch apart your ribs and hips.

2. Using momentum only at first, swing your right arm and leg up to begin warming up the hamstring. Use the opposite hand to check that your belly is concave. (Figure 1)

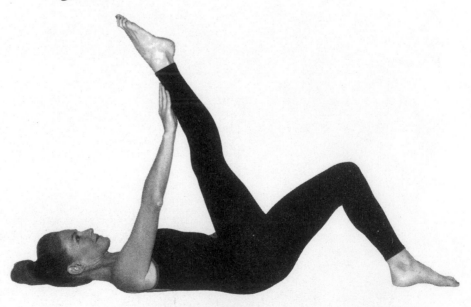

Figure 1

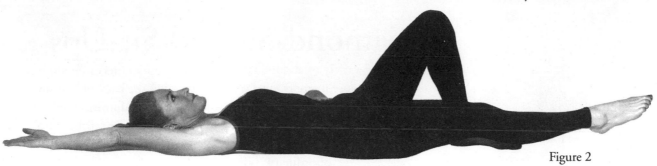

Figure 2

3. Lower and pull apart your right arm and leg to an inch from floor and repeat. (Figure 2)

4. On the fifth swing, hold back of thigh. Lightly place right hand behind thigh and left hand behind calf. Gently press in toward you as though the hamstring were a rubberband.

5. Now, let's get muscle specific for lengthening and strengthening: Flex your foot and begin a series of eight relax-and-contract motions where you bend the knee slightly for 1 to 2 seconds and then straighten for 3 to 4 seconds. Do not lock the back of the knee. Keep your heel slightly higher than your toes. (Figure 3)

6. On last strengthener, point and flex foot as you lower leg to the floor in 8 seconds. Then drop it, wobble, and relax.

7. Hug your knees, change legs, and repeat.

Recovery: Leg Shake

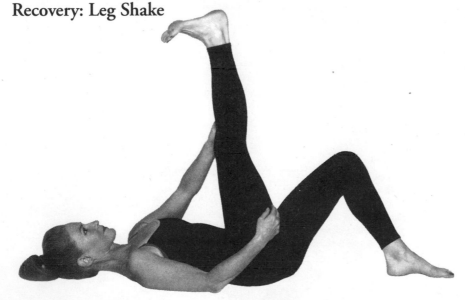

Figure 3

> ## Your Muscle Memory Voice
> ➤ *Is there a long space between my ear and shoulder? Between my ribs and hips?*
> ➤ *Is my pubic bone pulling up and tail bone tilting down?*
> ➤ *Are my leg muscles balanced so my knee is aligned and not stiff?*

Hamstring Muscles Reflect the Level of Tension in the Body

They can get tense from a day of driving or sitting at a desk. To prevent this, flex and move your knee around to feel the quadriceps on front and hamstring on back working evenly. This keeps your knees balanced and not locked. Do the Hamstring Strengtheners right in your bed if you wake up feeling stiff or before going to sleep after a tense day.

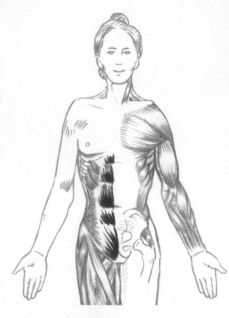

Primary Muscles Used:

Rectus and Upper Abdominals

Muscle: Rectus abdominis
Origin: Pubic bone
Insertion: Breast bone

Muscle: Obliques
Origin: 5th through 8th ribs
Insertion: Center of belly

Muscle: Serratus
Origin: 1st through 9th ribs
Insertion: Shoulder blade

Diamond-Shaped Sit-Ups

Among the variety of abdominal crunches and curls, I recommend this exercise because it works great without straining the back or stressing the neck and shoulders. Squeezing both the **rectus abdominis** (runs up and down the front of your belly) and **oblique** muscles (at the side, within your ribs and pelvis), gives you *double* the workout of ordinary abdominal exercises.

Number
Start with five, work up to ten.

Position
Lie flat on your back with arms stretched over your head, keeping knees slightly bent. Tighten belly and relax neck and shoulders.

Breathing
Inhale as you lift. Exhale when you roll up and lean forward.

Instructions
1. Lift your head and shoulders and swing your arms forward. (Figure 1)
2. Squeeze the **rectus** and **serratus** muscles and slowly curl straight up, arms reaching up. Knees slightly bent to equalize torso and leg length. (Figure 2)
3. Open knees into diamond shape with the bottoms of feet touching.

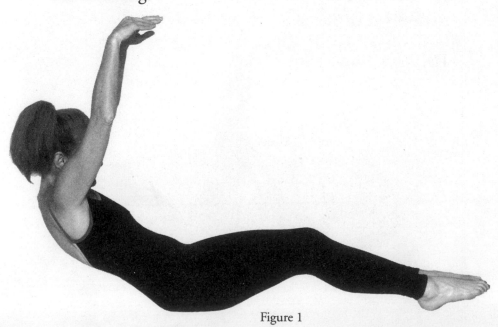

Figure 1

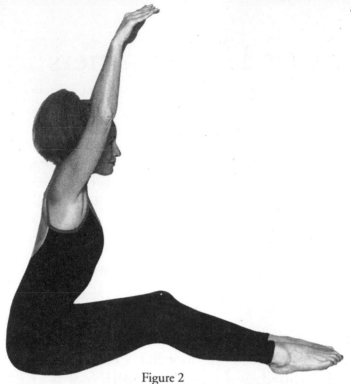

Figure 2

4. Dropping head and shoulders, bend forward. Stretch from under buttocks, pull in belly and feel lower back muscles strengthen and relax. (Figure 3)

5. Squeeze the **oblique** muscles in and return to a sitting position, rib cage lifted and arms reaching up. Keep knees softly bent and legs together. (Figure 2)

6. Roll back down slowly, back rounded and belly pulled in hard. Remember to keep knees slightly bent.

Recovery Stretch: Leg Shake

The Bonus Benefits of the Diamond-Shaped Sit-Ups

Squeezing in at the front of your ribs and hips helps make your body more narrow and prevents a "middle-age spread." Knowing where the waist muscles are, you can re-train them throughout the day to stay pulled in and give your belly that flat, concave look.

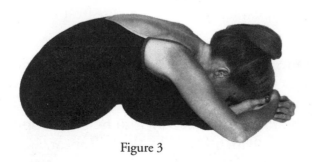

Figure 3

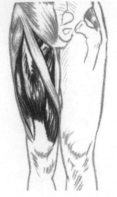

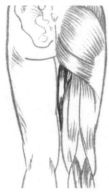

Primary Muscles Used:

Adductors and Quadriceps

Muscle: Adductors
Origin: Pubic bone
Insertion: Thigh bone

Muscle: Quadriceps
Origin: Top of thigh bone
Insertion: Knee cap

Note: At any point during this exercise that it stops being merely hard and may start to become irritating, stop and rest. Bring the knee in towards your chest, turn it out to the side and rest the foot on opposite knee.

Inner-Thigh Firmers

It takes only two minutes of concentrated effort per leg to complete this inner-thigh regimen which will definitely make your jeans fit better! Count your movements out loud to help you breathe and prevent boredom. Don't just use momentum—imagine you're lifting with an extra weight on your inner thigh to get really firm. Remember to keep kneecap unlocked throughout the exercise. At the end of the instructions, you'll find an alternate Inner-Thigh Firmer that may feel more comfortable.

Number

For each way, start with four repetitions, work up to eight for each way, then work up to thirty-two. It helps to count the thirty-two repetitions in four sets of eight!

Position

Sit on floor, right knee bent, foot flat. Left leg straight down, slightly lifted, and turned out, with foot flexed. Lean back on elbows. Keep belly pulled in with your neck and shoulders relaxed. (Figure 1)

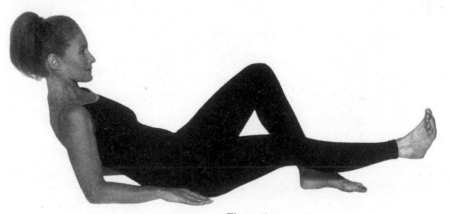

Figure 1

Breathing

Breathe naturally, exhaling during the greatest effort.

Instructions

FIRST WAY. Squeeze in **adductor muscles** along inside of thigh. Intensify the exercise by using these muscles, which face the ceiling, as the motor that lifts the leg. With legs pressed together, slowly raise left leg to height of opposite knee and lower to 1 inch from the floor. Repeat.

SECOND WAY. Begin with leg next to bent knee. Do little 2-inch lifts up and down near knee. Repeat. (Figure 2)

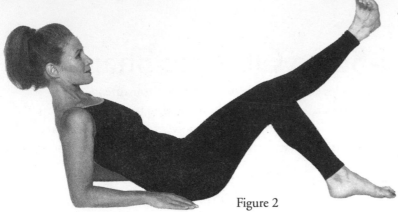

Figure 2

Your Muscle Memory Voice

➤ *Am I pulling my ribs in front down and lifting the ribs in back?*
➤ *Is my pubic bone pulling up and tail bone tilting down?*
➤ *Are my leg muscles balanced so my knee is aligned and not stiff?*

THIRD WAY. Begin with leg next to bent knee. Bend slightly, then squeeze inner thigh muscles to straighten leg. Repeat.

FOURTH WAY. (New position: Keep right knee bent, foot flat. Lift left leg straight up, parallel, and pressed next to bent knee.) Squeeze **quadriceps** on front of thigh to slowly bend and straighten the lower part of left leg. (Figure 3)

Do entire series with right leg.

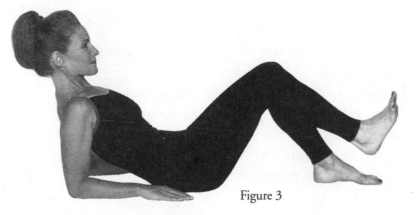

Figure 3

Recovery Stretch: Turned-Out Hip Relaxer

ALTERNATIVE EXERCISE:

Position
Lie on right side with right leg extended and left knee bent in front of body on a straight line with hip. Keep foot down and knee either on the floor or tilted towards ceiling, whichever feels more comfortable. Bend right arm and rest head on elbow. Keep spine straight.

Instructions
1. Flex foot and slowly lift and lower right leg a few inches from floor eight times. Increase to four sets of eight times.
2. Repeat with toes pointed eight times. Increase to four sets of eight times.
3. Alternately point and flex foot as you lift and lower leg eight times.
4. Change sides and repeat. Keep belly pulled in tight so both hips stay stacked in a perfectly straight line.

Recovery Stretch: Turned-Out Hip Relaxer

Firm Your Thighs Throughout Your Day

Since we rarely isolate our inner thigh muscles in daily activities (unless we horseback ride!), to strengthen them, try this. Based on the theory that whichever muscle faces the ceiling is the one that lifts the body weight, when you're standing around, just turn one leg out slightly, flex your foot and do little lifts. You can turn empty time into fitness time!

Two-Stage Oblique Shapers

Loose clothing styles and the desire to feel comfortable often shift our focus away from the size of our waistlines. For appearance and function, we want the power of strong **oblique muscles** every time we twist from side to side in sports or other activities. This exercise targets the torso.

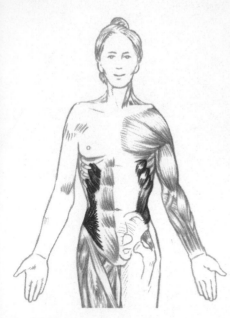

Primary Muscles Used:

Oblique and Transverse Muscles

Muscle: External oblique
Origin: Side of rib cage
Insertion: Top of hip

Muscle: Internal oblique
Origin: Lower hip
Insertion: Lowest ribs

Muscle: Transverse
Origin: Inside lowest ribs
Insertion: Across waist

Note: Because the direction of the oblique muscle fibers is diagonal, visualize a letter "**V**" from the pubic bone to the inside of the hips for the **internal obliques** and an upside down "**V**" from the sternum to the inside of the ribs for the **external obliques.** As you squeeze in, feel for cords at the side of the waist. The **transverse muscle** runs like an east-west cut along the waist.

Number
Ten times. Begin with Stage One. With increased strength, move to Stage Two.

Position
Lie on your back with your knees bent, feet flat on floor. Arms folded at the back of your head.

Breathing
Inhale as you're changing sides. Exhale as you "set" the muscle.

Instructions
Stage One

1. Bring right knee in towards chest with leg slightly lifted.

2. Raise from under head and shoulders, twist at waist and touch left elbow to outside of knee. Press against right elbow to help lift your body higher. Once up, let go of the help from your upper back muscles, and concentrate your effort into the oblique muscles. (Figure 1)

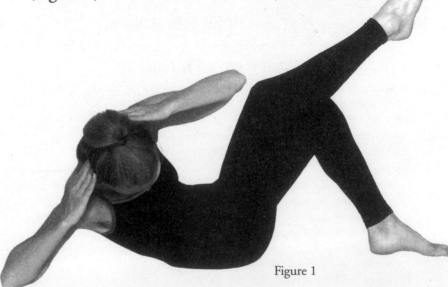

Figure 1

3. Lower your head to a few inches from floor and change sides.

4. After two changes, to lessen the help from your upper back muscles and isolate the obliques, keep the elbow back and lead more with your shoulder.

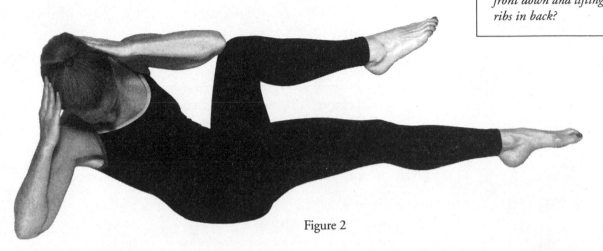

Figure 2

Stage Two

1. Identical to Stage One directions with one exception: keep the opposite, non-working leg straight and lifted 2 inches from the floor. Use leg to pull hip down. (Figure 2)

Your Muscle Memory Voice

➤ *Is there a long space between my ear and shoulder? Between my ribs and hips?*

➤ *Am I pulling my ribs in front down and lifting the ribs in back?*

Three Times the Benefit from the Two-Stage Obliques

Think of the ribs at the front, back, and sides of your torso whenever you're doing Oblique Shapers and you'll get three times the benefit. The **oblique muscles** function as a team and they stimulate your entire body in a chain reaction. Incorporate this thought into your daily moves. You'll regain awareness of your waist. When your torso has been still or your body's not warmed up, stand, turn, and use these muscles. This prevents back strain.

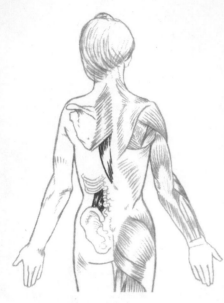

Primary Muscles Used:

Quadratus and Erector Spinae Group

Muscle: Quadratus lumborum
Origin: Back of pelvis
Insertion: Lower back
and last rib

Muscle Group: Erector spinae
(iliocostals, longissimus, spinalis)
Common Origin: Lower back
Common Insertion:
Ribs and neck

Note: Level One works well to strengthen your back muscles. As you use muscles to support the weight of your trunk, arms, and legs, they get stronger. I've added a second level for a little more interest and challenge because using an opposite arm and leg requires additional muscle strength to keep your balance. Build up back strength by keeping your abdominals pulled in very tightly and alternate between the two exercises.

Back Builders

Nature made our backs very strong with three layers of muscles to help protect the nerves, which emerge from the spine. Few people think about exercising their back muscles as much as the ones in front. Along with the abdominal muscles, the back muscles help support your trunk. And when fashion declares that "The Bare Back Is In," you'll be ready!

Number
Five times on each side. Begin with Level One; build up to Level Two.

Position
Begin on hands and knees, arms straight, spine straight, and back as flat as a table. Use all your back muscles to hold a straight line from neck to tailbone.

Breathing
Exhale as you round your back. Inhale as you straighten.

Instructions
Level One

1. Drop head down, squeeze in belly muscles, and round your back.

2. At the same time, bring right knee in towards chest, aiming to touch chest to thigh. (Figure 1: 1)

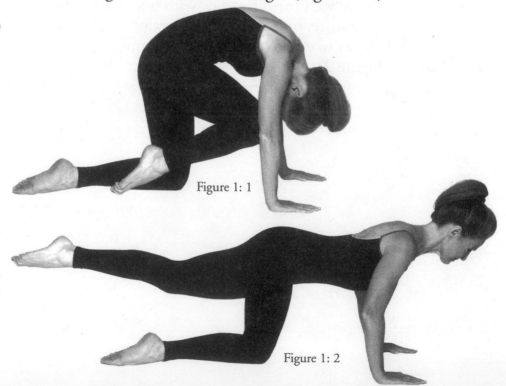

Figure 1: 1

Figure 1: 2

3. Lift tailbone to return to straight-back position. Soften elbows to allow spine to sink in between your shoulder blades.

4. At the same time, stretch right leg straight back on the same level as your back, making a straight line from ear to foot. (Figure 1: 2)

5. Repeat five times, sit back on heels to relax lower back. Change sides.

Figure 2: 1

Figure 2: 2

Level Two

1. As you round your back, bring your right knee and left elbow in, aiming to touch. (Figure 2: 1)

2. Straighten back, stretch right leg back and left arm forward at the same level as your back. Check alignment: Imagine a box beneath your hips which both sides touch. (Figure 2: 2)

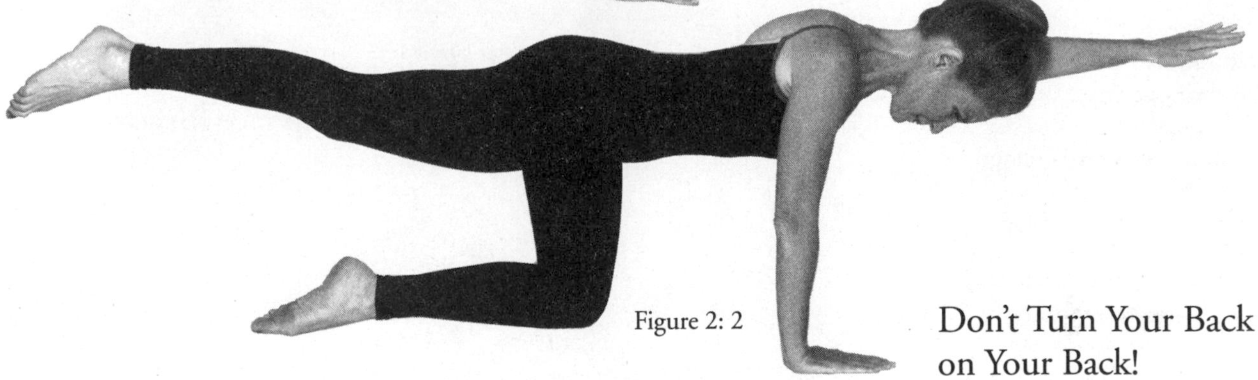

3. Repeat five times, sit back on heels to relax lower back. Change sides.

Recovery Stretch: Knee Pretzel

Your Muscle Memory Voice

➤ *Is there a long space between my ear and shoulder? Between my ribs and hips?*
➤ *Is the back of my head in a straight line with my upper back?*
➤ *Is my pubic bone pulling up and tailbone tilting down?*

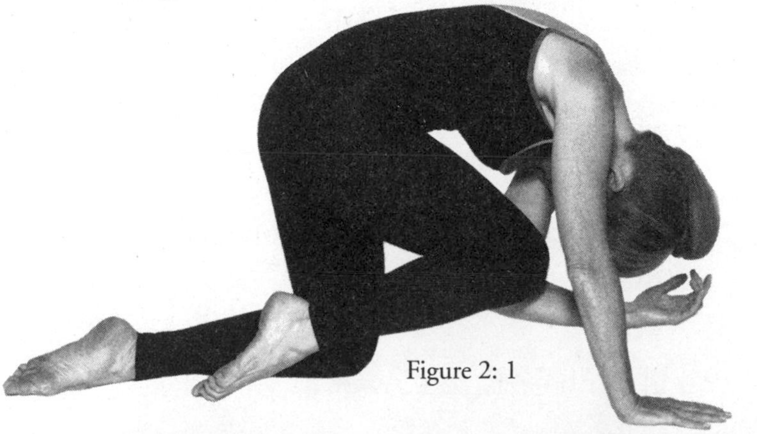

Don't Turn Your Back on Your Back!

The best way to keep your back healthy is to keep all the other muscles in shape because the back often does the work of a weaker muscle. When the belly is pulled in, the back automatically relaxes. Think of the vertical length of the **erector spinae muscles,** from the neck to the tailbone, and stretch apart your body so it looks and feels long and lean.

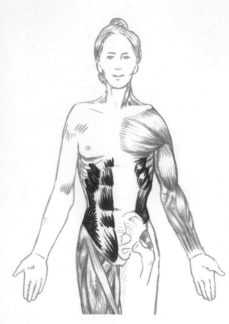

Lower-Belly Leg Lift

This looks like an exercise to firm the leg muscles
and it will. But we use it as the most effective way to isolate
and strengthen the lower abdominals. Your effort in
keeping the hip from moving as the leg raises and lowers is
what strengthens the abdominals. The muscles
stabilize the hips and pelvis.

Number
Twelve with each leg.

Position
Lie on right side in a completely straight line. Bend elbow
and rest head on arm. (Figure 1)

Breathing
Exhale as you lift. Inhale as you lower.

Instructions
1. Contract and pull in all the lower belly muscles.
2. Tighten thigh muscles. Knee and hip face forward.
   Keep your knee slightly bent.

Primary Muscles Used:

Lower Abdominals

Muscle: Rectus abdominis
Origin: Pubic bone
Insertion: Breast bone

Muscle: External oblique
Origin: Side of rib cage
Insertion: Top of hip

Muscle: Internal oblique
Origin: Lower hip
Insertion: Lowest ribs

Muscle: Transverse
Origin: Inside lowest ribs
Insertion: Across waist

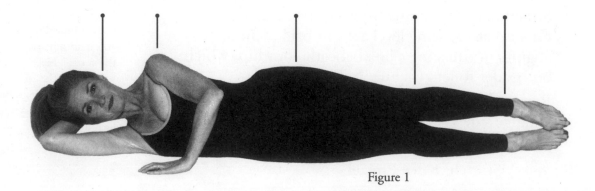

Figure 1

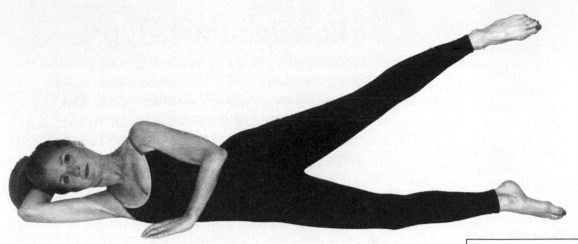

Figure 2

3. Slowly lift your left leg straight up, slightly higher than your hip. Imagine lifting with a heavy weight on your leg. Hold for three seconds and give the abductor muscles on your outer thigh an extra squeeze. (Figure 2)

4. Slowly press left leg down, using lower abdominals to keep hip still. Resist gravity's pull and lower leg to one inch from floor.

5. Take a few seconds after last lift for your body to memorize the feeling of straightness. Turn onto your back and repeat on the other side.

Your Muscle Memory Voice

➤ *Is the back of my head in the same line as my upper back?*
➤ *Am I pulling my ribs in front down and lifting the ribs in back?*
➤ *Is my pubic bone pulling up and tail bone tilting down?*
➤ *Are my leg muscles balanced so my knee is aligned and not stiff?*

All-Day Stomach Flattening

While sitting or standing, pull in your stomach as though you're closing a tight jeans zipper and an even tighter button. Pull in vertically, horizontally, and diagonally to draw in the muscles. A great tip for you: Squeeze the ligaments at the top of your inner thigh right alongside your pubic bone. This cordlike line in your groin works as you tighten your vaginal muscles to automatically contract the lower abdominals.

Positive Push-Ups

Strength—and the power that results from it—can be maintained with these push-ups. They strengthen your chest, shoulders, and arms. You'll always notice a woman who exercises this area by the firmness and vitality you see when she wears a v-neck or sleeveless shirt. Your body becomes the heavy weight, or "dumbbell," you use your arms to lift.

Number
Start with ten times. Work up to two sets of ten.

Position
Begin on hands and knees, arms straight. Place hands a bit more than shoulder-width apart, fingers pointed forward. Keep abdominals pulled in tightly. It is essential to keep good form: no drooping bellies or butts sticking up.

Breathing
Inhale as you lean forward. Exhale when you straighten arms.

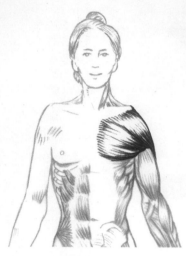

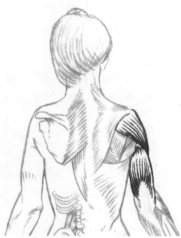

Primary Muscles Used:
Pectorals, Deltoids, and Triceps

Muscle: Pectorals
Origin: Shoulder bone
Insertion: First 7 ribs

Muscle: Deltoids
Origin: Top of shoulder
Insertion: Upper arm

Muscle: Triceps
Origin: Back of upper arm
Insertion: Elbow

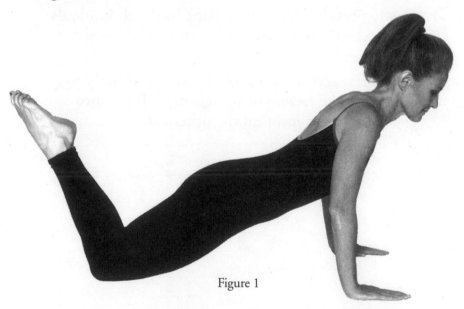

Figure 1

Your Muscle Memory Voice

➤ *Do I feel the same strength in my chest and upper back?*
➤ *Is my chest more forward than my belly?*
➤ *Can I drop a plumb line from the ceiling and have it go down the center of each body segment in a straight line?*

Instructions

1. Raise lower legs off floor either with feet parallel or ankles crossed. Lean body forward diagonally to form a straight knee-to-ear line. (Figure 1) (For beginners: Round your back and keep lower legs on floor.)

2. Bend elbows and lower hips as low as you can, keeping your body in a straight line. Stop just above the floor.

3. Straighten elbows and "push" the weight of your body up.

4. Repeat ten times. Sit back on heels and relax after ten. Work up to two sets of ten.

Recovery Stretch: Knee Pretzel

Positively Reinforce the Positive Push-Ups

After you're familiar with the feeling of the **triceps muscle** tightening, here's something to do during the day: Keep your shoulder pointed straight towards the ceiling and completely still, and rotate your arm in (thumb turns back). You can do this with arms down by your side or stretched horizontally at shoulder level to feel the muscle tone along the back of your arm.

Note: A standing version puts less stress on your wrists and arms. Place your hands on a wall at shoulder level. Stand arms-length away from the wall, with feet hip-width apart.

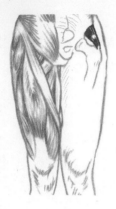

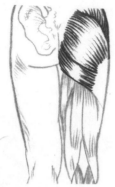

Sexy Bun Lifters

The buttocks muscles are the largest ones in your body. They can also be the most attractive. They may drop with age and a sedentary lifestyle but can be tightened and lifted effectively with this standing exercise. You gain the added benefit of firming your thighs while you raise your butt.

Number
Start with one set of ten, work up to forty. It helps to count the forty repetitions in four sets of ten!

Position
Stand with feet shoulder-width apart, hands on hips, weight toward the balls of feet.

Breathing
Inhale as you lower. Exhale as you lift.

Primary Muscles Used:

Gluteus Maximus, Medius, and Minimus

Muscle: Gluteus maximus
Origin: Hip and tailbone
Insertion: Thighbone

Muscle: Gluteus medius
Origin: Hip
Insertion: Thighbone

Muscle: Gluteus minimus
Origin: Hip
Insertion: Hip joint

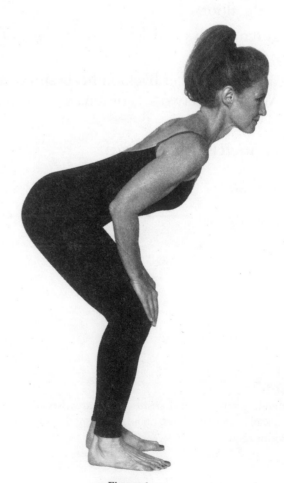

Figure 1

Instructions

1. Bend knees and lower body half way down as though sitting back on a chair. Place hands lightly on knees. (Figure 1)

2. Stay down, lift tailbone high, and flatten back.

3. Squeeze buns together tightly and keep back flat until almost standing.

4. Holding stomach in and buns tight, stand up slowly. (Figure 2)

5. Walk around. Lift and shake one leg at a time to recover.

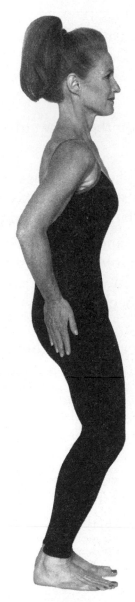

Figure 2

Your Muscle Memory Voice

➤ *Is my chest more forward than my belly?*
➤ *Is my pubic bone pulling up and tail bone tilting down?*
➤ *Are my leg muscles balanced so my knee is aligned and not stiff?*
➤ *Are my feet balanced? Is the center of my body directly above my arches?*

Daily Bun-Lifting Tips

Loss of muscle power in the thighs can be prevented with this exercise and by walking up and down stairs when convenient. We need strong thighs for most activities. When you stand, use your strong gluteal muscles to keep your butt lifted. When sitting, keep your chest in front of the belly by slipping the edge of a paperback book (about ½-inch thick) underneath the bottom of your hip bones. This will prevent the weight from pressing down into and spreading the buttocks.

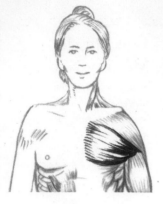

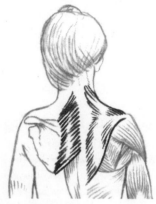

Primary Muscles Used:

Pectorals, Rhomboids, and Trapezius

Muscle: Pectorals
Origin: Shoulder bone
Insertion: First 7 ribs

Muscle: Rhomboids
Origin: Spine of middle back
(underneath trapezius)
Insertion: Shoulder blade

Muscle: Trapezius
Origin: Spine of middle back
Insertion: Collar bone

Shoulder Circles

Don't be fooled by how simple this exercise looks.
By concentrating and feeling the stretching and tightening of
the specific muscles, you'll be able to hold yourself straight
all the time. This exercise is one of the foundations of Muscle Memory.
When your chest, upper back, and neck muscles are strong,
you can engage them whenever you feel yourself slumping. You'll
also prevent that round-shouldered look.

Number
Ten times.

Position
Stand with feet hip-width apart. Keep belly pulled in,
chest in front of stomach, and head and upper back
in a straight line.

Breathing
Inhale to begin. Exhale on the backward circle.

Instructions
1. Bend your arms and place your fingertips on
   shoulders. Keep your shoulders pointed towards the
   ceiling and tip them farther back than your elbows.
2. Lift shoulders slightly and make a slow circling
   motion behind you. Hold for three seconds and feel
   the **pectoral** muscles on your chest lengthen as you
   push your shoulders back.
3. Keep shoulders back and pull down. Feel the shoulder
   blades come together as the **rhomboids** are tightening.
   (Figure 1)
4. Repeat ten times.
5. Drop arms, wobble head, and shrug shoulders to relax.

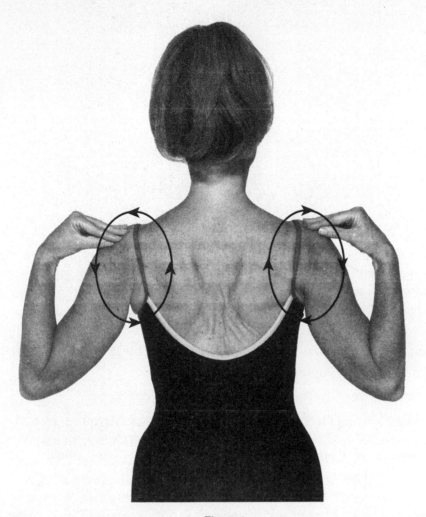

Figure 1

Your Muscle Memory Voice

➤ *Is there a long space between my ear and shoulder? Between my ribs and hips?*
➤ *Is the back of my head in the same line as my upper back?*
➤ *Do my shoulders point straight to the ceiling?*
➤ *Do I feel the same strength in my chest and upper back?*
➤ *Am I pulling my ribs in front down and lifting the ribs in back?*
➤ *Is my chest more forward than my belly?*
➤ *Is my pubic bone pulling up and tail bone tilting down?*
➤ *Are my leg muscles balanced so my knee is aligned and not stiff?*
➤ *Are my feet balanced? Is the center of my body directly above my arches?*
➤ *Can I drop a plumb line from the ceiling and have it go down the center of each body segment in a straight line?*

The Way to a Flatter Stomach Begins at the Shoulders

This may seem surprising, but when the head and shoulders stay lifted, you are more easily able to contract your stomach. Gravity is known to pull everything down. But now, with upper body strength, use Muscle Memory to hold yourself straight up against gravity. The ribs will stay lifted out of the hips and your stomach will look flatter.

Recovery Stretches

I have translated the instinctive movements we make to feel better after exercise into structured "recovery" stretches. We naturally shake our legs out, stretch our arms up, bend our necks in different directions, and do other similar motions to relax. You already unconsciously know how to "recover." But these three stretches are very muscle and joint specific.

HUGGING IS GOOD FOR YOU

I remember a bumper sticker that used to say, "Have you hugged your child today?" A little personal touch can help release tension.

If you ever feel strain in your lower back muscles, simply lie down on your back or side, bring one or both knees in towards your chest, and hug them. For upper back stiffness, hug your shoulders. And if you happen to be sitting in a small space for a while, stand up and do the same things.

Here are three Recovery Stretches. After some of the Daily Ten exercises, I've suggested you use one of them. But they're yours to use whenever you need them.

Leg Shake

As we elevate our legs in this exercise, we eliminate stiffness and improve our circulation, as well. Elevating the legs higher than the level of the heart uses the gravitational pull to help drain excess fluid from them. It's fun to just let go and shake.

Position
Lie on your back, knees bent, with belly pulled in and neck and shoulders relaxed throughout the exercise.

Instructions
1. Bring knees in towards chest, hug and circle them three times in each direction. (Figure 1)
2. Stretch legs towards ceiling. Place hands lightly on back of thighs. Touch your muscles to increase your focus.
3. Wobble all your leg muscles and shake vigorously. Feel your knees loosen and your feet get floppy. (Figure 2)
4. At first, shake for ten seconds, bend your knees, and repeat. Work up to about a minute, or until your feet feel tingly.
5. Shake for as long as you can, then bend your knees, hug them, and relax.

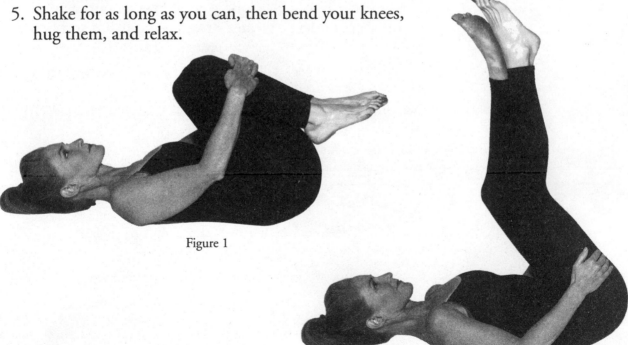

Figure 1

Figure 2

Turned-Out Hip Relaxer

Think of the construction of a hip joint and how the top of the thigh bone fits smoothly into the socket of the hip. With this in mind, you are able to rotate your thigh and release the muscles in the area to maintain your hip flexibility. You can do this as a restful position or an active stretch.

Position
Lie on your back with knees bent, feet flat on floor.

Instructions
1. Bring your right knee in towards your chest, turn it out, and rest that foot on or near the opposite knee. (Figure 1)

2. Keep foot on thigh, slide it towards you and massage it. Press thumbs along bottom of foot, near your metatarsal arch, pushing up and in. Use fingers to stretch apart the top.

3. Lift knees in this position, hold on, and bring them closer in towards you. When you hold behind your thighs, you get a greater release in the hip. (Figure 2)

4. Either keep your head and shoulders relaxed and down on the floor, or lift and aim forehead towards knee. Keep belly pulled in, a long space between your ear and shoulder and feel a greater stretch in your hip and back.

5. Bring knees in towards chest, lift legs, and shake.

6. Repeat on other side.

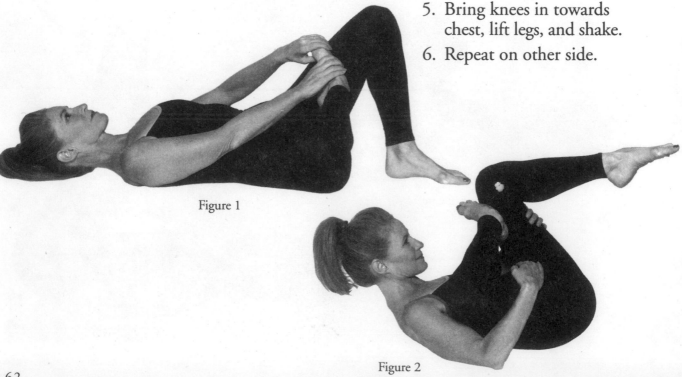

Figure 1

Figure 2

Knee Pretzel

The hip and spine are very responsive to stretching in this position. You exhale and use your body weight to follow the downward direction of gravity, which increases the stretch. Even though your body gets twisted and turned, you'll feel very stable and relaxed.

Position
Begin on hands and knees, elbows relaxed.

Instructions
1. Keep toes down as you stretch right leg straight back and across, all the way towards the left. (Figure 1)

2. With knees close together and feet very wide apart, sink back towards the floor. (Figure 2)

3. Pull in your belly. Use your breath and the weight of your body to feel the hips and spine release. For a greater stretch in your right hip, keep both hips down, hold on to your knees, and twist the ribs and spine in the other direction.

4. Raise up to your hands and knees, sit back on your heels, and sway from side to side to relax.

5. Repeat on other side.

ALTERNATIVE STRETCH:

If you are not comfortable in the hand-and-knee position, you can substitute this alternate Knee Pretzel and achieve similar results.

Instructions
1. Lie on back and bring knees in towards chest.
2. Cross right knee over left, exhale, and sink knees towards the left side.
3. Turn rib cage towards right and look beyond your shoulder.
4. Bring knees back to center and repeat on the other side. Be sure to keep head and shoulders relaxed and down on floor.

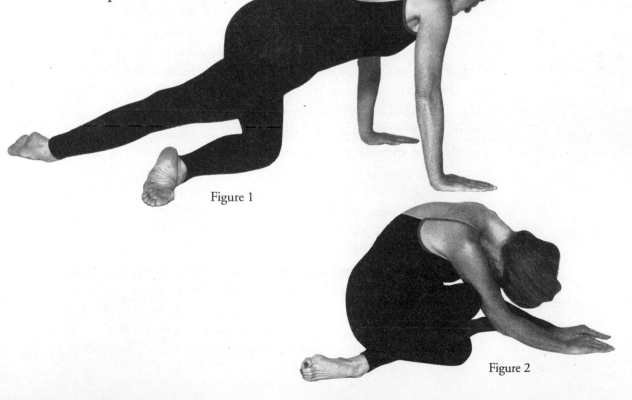

Figure 1

Figure 2

MAXIMIZING YOUR RESULTS

You have just taken ten giant steps toward a lifetime of fitness and health. Each of the Daily Ten has a specific purpose and can become deeper and more personalized whenever you practice it. When you practice anything every day, you know you'll improve at it.

Remember...

Start each exercise slowly in a warm-up mode. When your body feels comfortable, increase the intensity.

Customize the exercise. When you understand what each exercise is supposed to accomplish, you'll be able to customize it for your own body. You can achieve the same results as long as you work the same targeted body part.

Be muscle specific. You're doing fewer repetitions so make each one count by keeping your focus constant and holding for those few extra seconds to "set" your muscle.

Maintain alignment. Moving your arms and legs affects your fundamental alignment. After learning the answers to the Muscle Memory Quiz, you will develop a mental image that will put you back into correct alignment.

Create a visual image. Visualize the fibers pulling together, and match that vision with the feeling in your muscle. Help your body respond by wiggling into the position as you hold your muscle. When I asked the class to pull in at the waist, one student said that she sews a lot and thinks of gathering in the waist from the side to the front, "as though I'm gathering in a length of cloth to make a ruffle." Create your own images for the different movements of the exercises.

Use momentum to start. Although it's correct to use momentum to get started, don't let it replace the individual work of a muscle. Let go of the help when you're in position.

Respect exercise as a medical prescription. Exercise is therapeutic; it is meant to be specific and heal. In the same way that you adhere to a doctor's medical prescription, follow the directions and recommendations carefully.

Change Old Habits

See if you have any structural habits that deter you from keeping your alignment straight. Now that you're learning how proper muscle usage feels, you may be surprised to discover that changing some habits will make a big difference. Are your feet or hips turned out? Is your pelvis tipped either too far forward or too far back? Do you lean toward or favor one side?

Maxims

1. Always use all the muscles on the front, back, and sides of your body.
2. Always be sure you know where each part of your body is.
3. Always keep joints relaxed.
4. Feel something working every time you move. Nothing is a throwaway.
5. Be sure the fundamental body (neck, shoulder, ribs, and hips) is in correct alignment when you work the extremeties (arms and legs).
6. Use the connection of the arms to the upper body and the legs to the lower body to get additional stretch and strength.
7. Take a couple of seconds at the end of each exercise for the body to memorize the feeling of straightness you will transfer to standing up.

Keep in mind the gridlike intersecting body planes we discussed in Chapter Two. Let the Daily Ten exercises and your Muscle Memory Voice help you retrain your body to match them.

FIVE-MINUTE WORKOUT	FIVE-MINUTE WORKOUT	FIVE-MINUTE WORKOUT
Lower-Belly Leg Lifts	Sexy Bun Lifters	Back Builders
Diamond-Shaped Sit-Ups	Inner-Thigh Firmers	Positive Push-Ups
Neck Lengtheners	Hamstring Strengtheners	Two-Stage Oblique Shapers
Shoulder Circles	Shoulder Circles	Shoulder Circles

Five, Five, and Five

The Daily Ten exercises are meant to be done all at once in fifteen minutes. But you can still achieve benefits by dividing them into three five-minute workouts each day. Take five minutes in the morning, five minutes right before a meal or after a meeting, and five minutes before bed to take care of your muscles.

Separate the workout by selecting exercises that target each of your body segments. You can always tell where your clothes feel too tight. Do the Shoulder Circles not only with every five-minute segment but a few times during the day to counteract all the forward motion in our lives.

Listen to Your Muscle Memory Voice

For the first few weeks, remind yourself to train your Muscle Memory Voice. After a while your new habits will become your usual habits and be easy to maintain.

Correct posture becomes second nature with the Muscle Memory Method. This doesn't mean that you always sit and stand at attention. It means that every time your mind and body remember the good form your muscles achieved during exercise, you'll automatically make the necessary adjustments. When you catch your reflection in a store window, notice your alignment and apply your Muscle Memory Voice to improve it. If you're slumping forward at your desk or sitting on a bleacher at a baseball game, the moment you notice you're hunching, you'll sit up straighter, pull in your abdominals, move your head back, and look straight.

Your Muscle Memory Voice will become your best inspirational friend.

You Are Brilliant

From the first moment you picked up this book and decided to try to make a commitment to simple, intelligent exercise, you were brilliant. You don't have to wait to "get it right" to be brilliant. You don't have to wait to call yourself brilliant until your alignment is perfect. You are brilliant now because you have the power and the ability to be lean, strong, flexible, and healthy for the rest of your life.

Make this program a powerfully personal one between your mind and body.

MUSCLE MEMORY MAGIC

Questions and Answers

On the following page, you will find the complete Muscle Memory Quiz. Make copies and put them everywhere! Answering the ten questions puts into play everything you've learned. The muscles used in each of the exercises are used again in order to answer the Quiz correctly.

This is the value of Muscle Memory. You will always be in shape as long as you hear your Muscle Memory Voice and remind yourself to take the Muscle Memory Quiz.

THE MUSCLE MEMORY QUIZ

1. Are there two long spaces in my body: Between my ear and shoulder? Between my ribs and hips?

2. Is the back of my head in the same line as my upper back?

3. Do my shoulders point straight to the ceiling?

4. Do I feel the same strength in my chest and upper back?

5. Am I pulling my ribs in front down and lifting the ribs in back?

6. Is my chest more forward than my belly?

7. Is my pubic bone pulling up and tail bone tilting down?

8. Are my leg muscles balanced so my knee is aligned and not stiff?

9. Are my feet balanced? Is the center of my body directly above my arches?

10. Can I drop a plumb line from the ceiling and have it go down the center of each body segment in a straight line?

Here are the words to help your muscles and body "answer" the Muscle Memory Quiz. Do this during the exercises. Then do it any time, in any position you'd like. Think about taking it everywhere you go. As often as you want to, whenever the mood strikes, and especially when a tensed-up neck catches your attention, here is how to get instant alignment and all-day fitness.

This quiz is three parts mental and one part physical. For each of the ten Muscle Memory Quiz questions, I'll:

1. Show you how to check without a mirror that you're moving your body into the correct position.

2. Review the primary muscles used in holding the position.

3. Refer you to the exercise from the Daily Ten that established the Muscle Memory Voice you use for each answer.

The one part physical is already in your body—from the Daily Ten Muscle Memory Workout!

Answers to
the Muscle Memory Quiz

1. **Are there two long spaces in my body: Between my ear and shoulder? Between my ribs and hips?**

   Ear and Shoulder: Use your hands to check for long spaces. Spread the fingers on one hand. Put thumb at tip of shoulder and third finger at ear lobe.

   As you stretch and lengthen the **trapezius muscle** across the upper back and neck, move your head up so the finger no longer connects to the ear lobe.

   Neck Lengtheners

   Ribs and Hips: Press third finger into top of hip and thumb on back of ribcage. Feel the definition at your waist.

   With your abdominals pulled in, use the **latissimus** across the middle back and think of lifting from the back of your waist.

   Back Builders

2. **Is the back of my head in the same line as my upper back?**

   Hold a ruler, a piece of paper, or your hand vertically on the upper back. Move it up and see that your head touches it.

   Using the turning part of the exercise that strengthens the **sternocleidomastoid** (the long strip of muscle at the side of your neck), wobble your head and position it in a straight line with the upper back.

   Neck Lengtheners

3. **Do my shoulders point straight to the ceiling?**

   Visualize a vertical line going from the tip of your shoulders straight up towards the ceiling. Check that your shoulder does not roll forward.

   Keeping the ribcage and head lifted, spread out the **pectorals** in front and use the **trapezius** in back to hold the shoulders back and down.

   Shoulder Circles

4. **Do I feel the same strength in my chest and upper back?**

   Wobble your shoulders, and as the **pectorals** on the chest start working, feel the spine sinking in between the shoulder blades.

   As the pectorals stretch out and lengthen, they also strengthen as do the **rhomboid muscles** which pull the shoulder blades together.

   Positive Push-Ups

5. **Am I pulling my ribs in front down and lifting the ribs in back?**
With your thumbs in back and fingertips in front, tilt forward and backward. Feel the ribs in front pointing down on the diagonal and the back lifting. Notice how every time you move the front of your rib cage, the back also moves and vice versa.

   Lightly grasp the inner border of ribs in front and use the **rectus muscle** to pull them in and down in the same way you would close the buttons and tuck in a very tight shirt. The **latissimus** in back lifts the rib cage right out of the hips.
Diamond-Shaped Sit-Ups

6. **Is my chest more forward than my belly?**
Place one hand lightly across breasts. Slide it down towards the hips and don't let your belly touch the hand.

   Squeeze in at the waist and use the **oblique muscles** to pull your rib cage forward. Relax across the back of the waist. Slide your hands down from the side of your ribs and position them directly over the hips.
Two-Stage Oblique Shapers

7. **Is my pubic bone pulling up and tail bone tilting down?**
With your thumb at the belly button and third finger on your pubic bone, check for a short space between both points. Now place the thumb on the back of your waist and third finger on the tailbone trying to increase that space.

   Pull in and squeeze your **vaginal, lower oblique,** and **rectus muscles** to feel a concave belly. Be aware of your lower back muscles relaxing and lengthening.
Lower-Belly Leg Lifts

8. **Are my leg muscles balanced so my knee is aligned and not stiff?**
Think of how it feels when you're holding your breath and the ribs stiffen. Avoid this feeling in the back of your knees to keep them easy and relaxed.

   Use the **quadriceps** on front and **hamstrings** on back to flex the knees. Visualize the same size, shape, and strength of both muscle groups.
Hamstring Strengtheners
Inner-Thigh Firmers

9. **Are my feet balanced? Is the center of my body directly above my arches?**
Wobble your feet forward and backward, inward and outward. Draw two imaginary lines across the front and back and the left

and right side of each foot. Your feet are balanced when those two lines intersect. Position the rest of your body so the center of your pelvis is directly above this point.
Sexy Bun Lifters

10. Can I drop a plumb line from the ceiling and have it go down the center of each body segment in a straight line?

If you were to suspend a plumb line from the ceiling, it would drop down in a straight, 180-degree line. To align the outside of your body, concentrate on your inside as you straighten.

Organize yourself from the bottom up. In the same way that a building needs a solid foundation before the roof is put on, balance your feet and pull up through the center of each of your body segments. Wobble around and stack them directly on top of each other.

Which exercises establish the physical power to accomplish a correct answer to Muscle Memory Quiz question 10?
All exercises from the Daily Ten Muscle Memory Method Workout!

THE ONE-MINUTE MUSCLE MEMORY BOOST

This boost does not stay within the boundaries of exercise. It never stops. It is your key to drawing on the power of everything you and your muscles learned from the Daily Ten Muscle Memory Workout and the Muscle Memory Quiz.

Use one minute when you only have a minute. Settle yourself and prepare for your next moment.

1. Pump your feet and legs for a strong foundation. Stand with your body feeling vital and correctly aligned.

2. Roll your shoulders back—one at a time—then hold both of them back.

3. Clasp both hands lightly together behind your back and, in this position, roll both shoulders farther back and pull them down. The work comes from the upper back and chest muscles, not your arms.

4. Be sure your shoulders point to the ceiling. Hold and "set" for a count of three.

5. Release your hands but keep pulling your shoulders down and stretch beyond your fingertips.

6. To complete the boost, position the back of your head in line with your upper back and keep stretching.

7. Breathe in deeply. As you exhale fully, take leave of the position. Your muscles will remember to keep the boost!

SAMPLE PROGRAM

As an approach to fitness that relies on your own intelligence, this program is yours to customize. One way of doing it is outlined below.

In Chapter Four you'll find the Five-Minute Stretch and Joint Loosener to help you maintain flexibility and the Three-Minute Breathing Relaxation. Chapter Five gives you Strength Training to Increase Bone Density and Shape Muscles. In Chapter Six, I'll outline my Intelligent Walking Program for Cardiovascular Fitness and Weight Management. And Chapter Seven offers three exercises to help you enhance your sexual pleasure.

You will always be in shape if you find a way to participate in all the aspects of this program over the course of your week. Decide if one week you'd like to concentrate on strength training a little bit more or whether you'd like to walk more frequently. When your mood or your schedule says "no exercise" then try a few Shoulder Circles and the One-Minute Muscle Memory Boost.

Remember, this is *your* program. Embrace and practice it for life.

**The Daily Ten Muscle
Memory Exercises** . . . . Six to seven days a week

Stretch and Joint Loosener . . . . Four to five times a week

Breathing Exercises . . . . Whenever you need them

**Strength Training to Increase
Bone Density and Shape Muscles** . . Three to four times a week

Intelligent Walking Program . . . . . . Three to six times a week

**Exercises for
Sensuality and Sexuality** . . . . As often as you like

---

Part Three

Joint Loosening, Stretching, and Breathing Exercises for Flexibility and Comfort

Our bodies have the potential to perform like well-oiled machines. We've reached adulthood and beyond, and our joints have accompanied us throughout this journey. Let's repay them in kind by giving them the attention they need.

This chapter shows you how to keep your body physically functioning for a long time. Practice loosening your joints to keep their full range of motion—or lose it.

FLEXIBILITY

Healthy joints enable us to move our necks, spines, arms, legs, hands, ankles, and even our mouths. Now, where would we be without that? Flexibility potential differs from person to person. Body type, genetic background, training, diet, and stress level all affect your flexibility. Your joints can ache when they are used beyond their capacity.

To see what I mean, try sitting on the floor with your legs stretched straight out in front. Now drop your head forward, round over, and see how close it comes to your knees. It will come close only if your top and bottom halves are equally flexible. The length of your legs in relation to your trunk determines the ease with which you can accomplish this. Here's how to help equalize the ratio if your legs are longer than your trunk: When you're doing exercises, bend your legs a bit to shorten them to match the length of your trunk. You can overcome an inherent lack of flexibility by strengthening and lengthening all your muscles.

Flexibility usually corresponds to your age level. But people who have healthy joints feel more comfortable and are less stiff than those who don't. Any time you can move a joint without experiencing pain, it's good for you. When you're exercising, if a joint feels tight and a bit hard to move, exercise slowly. But the moment it becomes irritating, stop.

Determine your current level of flexibility. You'll probably find you need to stretch more than you used to. You won't have to limit your activities, but you may want to reevaluate where you are at this point and whether what you're doing is comfortable and pleasurable. There is always a pleasurable level of intensity in which you can participate in any activity.

What Makes a Healthy Joint?

Once again, I am in awe of how brilliant a machine the body is. A joint is formed where the ends of two bones connect. At the beginning of our lives, the joint is a neat little package that's stable and flexible. Strong ligaments stabilize the joint and smooth joint linings keep us flexible. In the Joint Looseners, you're loosening all the connective tissue, muscles, and joints. Getting smarter about caring for our joints will slow down the wear-and-tear process.

Common joint problems can result from everyday use. Here's where correct alignment and muscle tone really come into play. The body is designed with vertical, horizontal, and coronal (front and back) planes. Joints stay healthy when these planes are equal. Picture the knee. When the thigh bone fits straight into the knee in a neutral, aligned position, there is equal pressure on the front and back of that joint. Having the same strength in your major thigh muscles—quadriceps on front and hamstrings on back—ensures an even balance. If, instead, you stiffen and force the knee back, there's more pressure in front and you'll wear the joint down unevenly. Arthritic changes can result from this kind of pressure and uneven rubbing on the bones.

Your best defense? Lessen the stress at every joint by aligning your bones and by stretching and strengthening the surrounding muscles to keep them in place. Have you ever noticed that the cups in your dinnerware break much more frequently than the plates? Those little handles on the side prevent them from being stacked straight. They're too unstable to counteract gravity.

Love Your Joints

Stretching is often neglected because it doesn't burn nearly as many calories as aerobics or weight training. People with time constraints and those concerned primarily with weight management usually choose a more vigorous activity. But after you do the exercises in this chapter, you'll want to keep that comfortable feeling in your joints.

Not only is each part of the body connected to another, there are also many similarities in the ways that they work. The movement of certain joints in the top half of the body parallels the movement of the joints in the bottom half. The hip and shoulder joints have a full range of motion and can move in many directions. Elbows and knees are hinge joints and can only bend up and down. Fingers and toes are so similar that if you had to, you could pick up a dropped napkin using your toes!

Physical comfort starts from deep within the body. What you see on the outside is a covering of the bony and muscular structures. With this program you'll zero in and understand which muscles do what and how they feel when they're working. Each component of the Muscle Memory Method program does something special for your body. But there are days when the only thing you may feel like doing are the Joint Looseners. Stretching and joint loosening lead to freedom in movement.

HEALTHY TIPS FOR PAIN-FREE SHOULDERS, BACK, AND HIPS

The Joint Loosening Exercises in this chapter are an excellent prescription against pain. Exercises are only part of the solution, however. It's using the muscles correctly all the time that will prevent pain. When correct usage is firmly established in your Muscle Memory, your alignment and bio-mechanics—the way you move—will be correct. Until then, remind yourself frequently to practice.

Tips like pulling in your belly to keep your back relaxed...rocking your knees to keep the hamstrings and quadriceps working evenly...breathing to release muscle stiffness caused by tension...moving to keep blood circulating through your muscles: These are all ways to avoid pain.

Non-specific pains and general stiffness are not necessarily the result of aging. They are your body's gracious way of calling attention to potentially serious problems. Continuous tension shortens and weakens muscles. The longer you hold a muscle, the more likely the body is to react with a defense mechanism that causes tightness and stiffness. This prevents the muscle from relaxing and pain can result. If you were to observe a working muscle in a physiology lab, you'd see that in order to maintain muscle flexibility and length, the muscle needs to relax and "let go" for the same amount of time it tenses and contracts.

When you're strengthening and toning, the action of tensing a muscle is what makes it stronger. The tensing of a muscle is also a normal response to nerve irritation. Unreleased tension gets stored up and disables muscles. This is one of the causes of pain. Nerves lie within and around the muscles and when the muscle becomes too tight or weak, it presses on and irritates the nerve.

Prevention is more desirable than trying to alleviate pain. One of the men who comes to my studio came, at first, only because his older tennis partner told him, "you want to play at seventy-nine? You better exercise your joints."

Shoulder Health

Stiffness occurs when the joint wrapping gets stiff. Certain occupations and normal body changes can cause joint stiffness. Many women tell me they are experiencing shoulder limitations and pains for the first time. The shoulder is extremely mobile but not very stable. Three bones meet at the shoulder: the collar bone, upper arm, and shoulder blade. Four small muscles in the shoulder's "rotator cuff" hold the ball part of the shoulder stable. Take a look at the anatomy chart on page 34 so that when you do the rotator cuff exercise you can be muscle specific. The four muscles—teres minor, supraspinatus, infraspinatus, and subscapularis—are a mouthful, but notice how small and intertwined they are. Feel them working, rather than the larger deltoid muscle that covers them. Pressure on the nerves in this area causes pain. This exercise will help prevent that.

Pain-Free Back

Your back stays healthy when the pelvis is aligned in the following neutral position: When the anterior and superior spines (front and back points on your pelvis) are in the same horizontal plane and the pubic bone and tailbone are in the same vertical line. This neutral alignment of the pelvis keeps the spine in the correct position. Too much or too little curve in the lower back causes pain.

A healthy back can bend in all directions but if you feel strain, only do the motions that feel comfortable. Try the Spinal Slide Joint Loosener or hug your knees.

Another major source of back pain is muscle imbalance. These exercises promote muscle balance, making back pain a condition you don't necessarily have to live with. When a muscle group is weak, other muscles must take over to do the job. This is often seen when people do abdominal (abs) exercises. You cannot raise your

A Simple Exercise to Strengthen Your Rotator Cuff

1. Stand with one arm bent in front at a right angle.
2. Turn it out to the side as though you are opening a door.
3. Place the other hand at the top of that shoulder to keep it still.
4. Return to starting position.
5. Repeat each side eight times slowly.

trunk and curl up with weak "abs." Instead, you rely on your back muscles to lift and this subjects you to pain.

Be aware that you have the use of your entire body for every task at hand. When you lift a heavy object, keep your back safe by bending your knees slightly and lifting with your legs. Keep the object close to your body and use strong abdominals to stabilize your spine.

Abdominals on the front protect the internal organs and stabilize the trunk, pelvis, and hips. We're all aware of them because we're concerned about our appearance. Muscles on the back support the spinal cord and often we don't think about them until we feel strain. Aside from their therapeutic value, back muscles are beautiful, too, and should be toned. The bare back is a classic fashion statement, whether in a bathing suit or in an evening gown. I tell my students, "what feels right therapeutically...looks right aesthetically."

Healthy Hips

We rely on our hips being healthy because we use them for so many activities. We address this area with the Joint Looseners and with the Recovery Stretches in Chapter Three. A group of muscles called the hip flexors need to be stretched to keep the pelvis aligned. Shortening of these muscles inhibits the ability to extend the hip joint and causes the lower back muscles to strain.

In the anatomy chart on page 34, you'll see muscles called adductors and abductors. Adduction and abduction describe the directions in which your body moves. Adduction is movement toward the body, and abduction is movement away from the body. The hip flexor group includes the psoas major, iliacus pectineus, adductors longus and brevis, rectus femoris, tensor faciae latae, and the sartorius.

The sartorius muscle, which goes from the hip to the knee, is the longest muscle in the body. You are said to have sartorial splendor when you are beautifully dressed and well-tailored. When you sit cross-legged, with your knees bent and one ankle over the other, it is called "tailor sitting."

Feel Comfortable and Healthy

The Joint Looseners help you get in touch with the natural way your body is meant to feel. You've been in your body for a long time. Who knows it better than you? If you feel stiff anywhere, move that area any way it feels good to move. Use Muscle Memory to help you direct your muscles.

The Sartorial Stretch

1. Either lie down or sit on the floor and lean back on your elbows.
2. Lift hip slightly, bend your knee, and turn it comfortably towards the center of the body.
3. Breathe in to the belly of the muscle and use your hands to feel the stretch along top of thigh.
4. Keep the other leg straight out on the diagonal, knee slightly bent and relaxed.
5. Repeat on other side.

Notice which habits you might change in order to feel more comfortable. Wearing a shoulder bag on one shoulder will definitely cause strain over time since you hike up your shoulder to keep the bag on. I try to wear a bag with a strap long enough to cross over my chest to have equal weight on both shoulders.

Knapsacks have now become popular in the United States for function and fashion. But so many people wear them only on one shoulder. Wear them as they're meant to be worn—on both shoulders.

Diet affects how our joints feel. In excess, sugar, caffeine, alcohol, and nicotine can be dehydrating and cause acidity. Bodies which have too much acid in their bloodstream level usually feel stiff. Experiment with lessening some of these dehydrating substances and see if this works for you. By cutting down on them and drinking plenty of water (about eight glasses a day), you can help the body's natural process of keeping the joints lubricated. Maintain hydration for every organ and cell in your body.

Feeling good means feeling comfortable and relaxed. One of the problems that can arise from a lack of muscle conditioning is cramping in the muscles. As your muscles become more conditioned, cramping will be less of a problem. But if it occurs, here's what you can do.

How to Avoid Muscle Cramps

We've been discussing how overuse can irritate your joints. Overuse and underuse similarly affect you and muscle cramps can occur in both situations. Most of you have felt your calves tighten up at one time or another and know how painful that can be. Remember that a muscle relaxes for the same amount of time it contracts and without that process, your muscle stays tense and can cramp.

Calcium, that necessary bone-building mineral, is also maintained in the blood level where it is used for muscle contractions. Calcium is stored during the day and lost at night. That's why grandmothers often said to drink a glass of warm milk before going to sleep. Lack of calcium is a major cause of muscle cramps. Water is essential to balance the smooth functioning of potassium and sodium. Some of my students find that taking quinine, either in pill form or in tonic water, will alleviate cramps. You can help avoid cramps with careful nutrition.

Use the following anti-cramping program whenever you need to. Remember to stretch to lengthen any shortened or tense muscles. Self-massage the tightened area to loosen tension and increase circulation to the area. Try to relieve the cramping by moving slowly, gently, and with awareness.

> ## HOW TO RELIEVE CRAMPS IN SPECIFIC PARTS OF YOUR BODY
>
> **In the Toes:** Rest the foot with cramped toes on opposite knee. Place fingers over toes and thumb under ball of foot. Fingers gently press toes down, thumb gently presses up.
>
> **In the Calves:** Standing, put palms against a wall at shoulder height. Place one foot about 12 inches from the wall, the other about 18 inches from the wall. Lean forward and bend the front knee. Lift and lower the back heel and feel the stretch in the back leg.
>
> **In the Shins:** Stand with feet crossed. Lean on outside edges of feet. Press the calf of one leg against the shin of the other. Breathe and hold for a count of three. Change sides.
>
> **In the Hamstring:** Pull your knee toward your chest. This automatically lengthens the muscle.
>
> **In the Upper Back:** Standing or lying down, cross arms over your chest, hold underneath shoulder blades, and hug yourself. Press your head down and keep a long line between your ear and shoulder.

Balanced, Centered, and Flexible

Your body can sense where all its parts are. Your *proprioceptors*—sensory receptors in the muscles, joints, and ligaments—will always help you maintain upright posture and stretch safely. The body senses changes and reacts using its automatic *stretch reflex*. Whether to counter the ongoing pull of gravity or to keep your balance in a tricky situation, you'll be ready. Proprioceptors send the balancing message to the spinal cord, which sends it to the muscles.

Good balance conserves energy and makes you feel confident, stable, and secure. There are times every day when being balanced prevents strain, injury, or a fall. With balanced muscles and an aligned body, Muscle Memory keeps you straight. This is done by integrating sensory input into the brain which then sends it to your muscles. When you don't have to fight gravity, look at all the muscle tension you're avoiding. You've moved effortlessly—you neutralized gravity.

Feeling balanced, visualize the center of your body where all the body planes intersect. Focus all your energy at the center to feel calmer and "centered." Throughout this program, we practice muscle balance. But balance can be thought of in psychological terms as well, as in feeling balanced. Balancing and centering have always been important in Eastern philosophies, based on being in harmony with nature. "Yin" and "yang" are naturally opposing but complementary forces in the universe. The female "yin" is passive, and represents the heavens, the moon, the night, and the autumn. Its symbol, the tiger, is unfathomable. The male "yang" is active and grounded, and represents the sun, the day, and the spring. Its symbol, the dragon, is assertive. We achieve our sense of balance when these forces work together. There are times when we can apply the "yin-yang" balancing principles and get through situations more easily. If life is in turmoil, try bringing your awareness right into your center, directly behind the navel. Connect your Muscle Memory Voice there and see if you can balance yourself.

My long-time colleague and friend, Edwige Gilbert, has brought this wonderful treat to the studio for the past twelve years.

EDWIGE'S BALANCING MEDITATION
*Breath represents life. Each breath is
a new beginning, a new possibility.*

Position
Stand with legs hip-width apart, knees slightly bent. Keep arms relaxed down by your side and feet planted firmly into the earth.

Instructions
1. Begin to imagine that long, deep roots are growing and growing underneath your feet, as if you had been magically transformed into your favorite tree. Feel its strength and begin to draw on the "yang" energy to provide yourself with a great sense of inner balance and inner connectedness. Dwell into this healing space for a moment.
2. Now switch your focus onto your spine. Keep standing where you are and imagine that an invisible, divine string attached to the top of your head is pulling you higher and higher towards heaven. Begin to feel lighter and lighter on your feet. Your body begins to tingle with "yin" energy and you experience an intense and growing feeling of well-being. Appreciate and smile into this miracle.
3. To conclude this powerful practice, slowly bring your hands, placed on top of each other, over your navel. As you hold them there, experience a current of heat flowing and circulating. This is a sign that "yin" and "yang" energies are perfectly blended together. Dwell into this moment, realizing it is the only moment.

Quietly Say to Yourself:
As I breathe in, I am energizing my body and my mind.
As I breathe out, I smile into this moment, which is the only moment, feeling loved.
I feel protected by a divine bright light that is circling all around me now.
May I experience love and joy in my life.
May I be free of pain and fear in my life.
May I discover compassion in my life.
May I awaken my potential and fulfill my destiny.
I surrender, body and soul, to this ultimate experience of peace within.

BEFORE WE BEGIN

Take the time to warm up muscles and loosen your joints before you use them. Warming up is different from stretching. You need to increase your body temperature and circulation before you can stretch. Never stretch an unused, cold muscle. For example, if you're playing a sport like tennis, practice the serving motion with your arm before you even toss the ball up to hit. Twist and bend your spine from side to side so it's ready for action.

Don't startle your body by reacting before it's ready to react. Try to get in the habit of moving your entire body, not just snapping your head or lurching forward. Turn to face a person who's speaking to you instead of just twisting your neck and upper back. Don't let tension accumulate by staying in one position for too long. Move around. Loosen up muscles that have held a phone or a steering wheel too long.

Let gravity work for you! When the focus is on Joint Loosening, I hold the stretching position longer and emphasize deep breathing. You allow your muscles and joints to relax and "let go" by breathing deeply. With additional breaths, you can go beyond the point where you felt restricted. Use the weight of your body along with the downward pull of gravity to get the greatest results.

Comfort and Flexibility

Now that you're familiar with the importance of healthy joints, you can actively contribute to your flexibility. Move each joint within its comfort zone several times a day. Try out different moves that feel good. Each joint has a natural range of motion. Start either at the top or bottom of your body. Roll, bend, or twist and—in a slow, quiet, and flexible way—loosen each part.

THE ANYTIME, ANYWHERE FLEXIBILITY PROGRAM

If you only have a few minutes to spare, you can do this program anytime, anywhere, just as you do your Muscle Memory.

For Your Neck: Tip ear to shoulder and circle head. Do not bend too far forward or back since this can be irritating. Use the Neck Lengthener from the Daily Ten to maintain a long, stretched neck with a space between the ear and shoulder.

For Your Shoulders: Do the Shoulder Circles from the Daily Ten. When strengthening the chest, shoulders, and upper back muscles, we do the Circles only in the backward motion since so many activities naturally roll us forward. But when flexibility is the goal, circle in both directions—backward and forward.

For Your Wrists: Make a loose fist and circle in both directions. Press your thumb against the cushion of each fingertip to stretch the forearm muscles.

For Your Torso: With hands on hips to feel stable, roll your torso in both directions, bend it from side to side, look over your shoulder, and twist. The rib cage connects directly to the spine and this is an efficient way to keep your spine flexible.

For Your Hips: Shift them from side to side; mimic a belly dancer's hip rolls.

For Your Knees: It's a hinge joint, so work it like one. Flex one foot and bend and straighten your knee.

For Your Ankles: With toes on floor, lift heel and circle in both directions.

The Program

You can take pleasure from becoming more flexible. As you loosen your joints, your movement abilities are enhanced and you feel more graceful. You may not have thought of movement only for movement's sake—movement not involved in a particular activity. Don't ignore your body, use and enjoy it. If you thought of yourself as someone who didn't like exercise, you may be surprised to discover that you do.

Do the five exercises on the following pages in whatever order your body feels like doing them. If you've taken exercise classes in the past, you may have heard a teacher say, "listen to your body." Sometimes you don't have to listen too hard. Your body will tell you loudly and clearly where it feels stiff or tense. Position yourself comfortably and move wherever you feel stiff.

People stretch in various ways, but everyone wants a method that is efficient and comfortable. In the fitness field, different methods have been popular over the years. I've used the following method for stretching muscles for many years with great results.

Stabilize the origin, move at the insertion, pull both ends in the opposite direction, feel the stretch in the belly of the muscle. Hold each stretch for three to four seconds, breathing into the belly of the muscle. Release the stretch for one to two seconds. Feel the opposing partner muscle. For example, during the hamstring stretch, feel the quadriceps working.

As you do the following exercises, think about the alignment principles. Free up tension and imagine a space between each joint. Your goal is flexibility but every time you use a muscle you tone it and strengthen your bones. Loosening helps you feel the difference between being tense and being relaxed. Learn this and you'll enjoy the relaxed feeling.

Breathing

Breathe in and out in a similar manner for all the exercises. Inhale as you begin your stretch and exhale into the belly of the muscle you're working. Hold the stretch until you feel the joint release and continue to breathe in a steady, slow rhythm.

Warming Up

Prepare for stretching and joint loosening with this simple warm-up exercise to increase the spaces in your body. It can be done standing up or lying down.

Standing, stretch one arm up, hold on to it with the opposite hand, and use the arm to pull up your rib cage. At the same time, bend one knee to pull the hip down. Check that your belly is in and you're not scrunching the shoulders. Keep a long space between the ear and shoulder.

Lying down on your back with knees bent, stretch one arm up and follow the standing directions. At the same time, lift one hip slightly and use the buttocks muscles to pull it down.

The Five
Joint-Loosening
Exercises

Spinal Slide

In addition to doing the spinal slide in your
Joint Loosening, you can also enjoy it in bed if you wake up stiff
in the morning. This is the best remedy whenever your back
feels stiff. You'll feel your back muscles and spine stretching. Visualize
a space between each of the twenty-four vertebrae. Bringing
the knee in toward your chest automatically tightens the abdominals
and stretches the back muscles. To begin warming up the shoulder,
add slow shoulder rolls on the last repetition.

Position
Lie comfortably in a sightly C-shaped position on one
side with an arm folded beneath your head. The lower
leg is slightly bent and the top leg rests on it.

Number
Three times each side.

Instructions
1. Raise top leg to level of hip. (Figure 1)

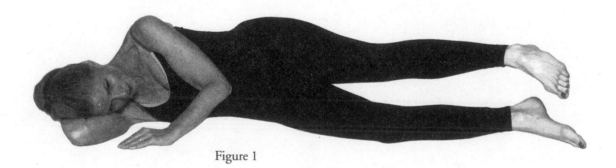

Figure 1

2. With hand behind thigh, gently bend knee towards chest, keeping abdominals pulled in. Curve your spine into a letter "C." Imagine pulling your belly button through your body so that it can emerge from the back of your waist. (Figure 2)

3. Slide leg back to starting position. Drop it and "let go" of muscle tension.

4. On the last repetition, bend the top arm and place fingertips on shoulder. Slowly prescribe three backward rolls. Feel the spine sinking in between the shoulder blades. Lengthen the lower back from the waist to the tailbone.

5. Hug knees, turn onto back, and repeat on other side.

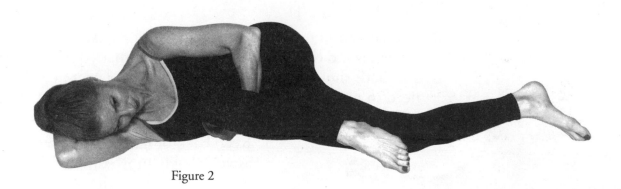

Figure 2

Shoulder and Hip Rotators

Both of these exercises—one for the shoulder and one for the hip—look and work the same way. Both joints are "ball and socket" joints, where a long bone fits into a groovelike socket and stretches in a full range of motion. Avoid using momentum. Use specific muscles to make the motion. Even though you're moving the arm or the leg, feel the loosening in the core of the joint.

...der and for the hip, imagine you are facing a clock and match each instruction to a specific number.

For the Shoulder

Position
Lie curled up on right side to stretch left shoulder. Keep your chest close to thigh, and forehead toward knee. Put right hand under top thigh and pull it in. Stretch left arm across body.

Number
Three times each side. Start slowly and increase the intensity as the joint loosens.

Instructions
1. Keep fingertips on floor and feel the ribs move as you stretch your left arm as far as you can, aiming towards the "9." (Figure 1)

2. Feel chest and upper back muscles working as you move toward the "12." Pause and check that your neck and both shoulders are flat against the floor. You may need to move the bent knee towards the ceiling in order to keep your fingers on the "12." (Figure 2)

3. Keep back of hand down now as you slowly move towards the "3" and end at the "6." The elbow stays slightly bent.

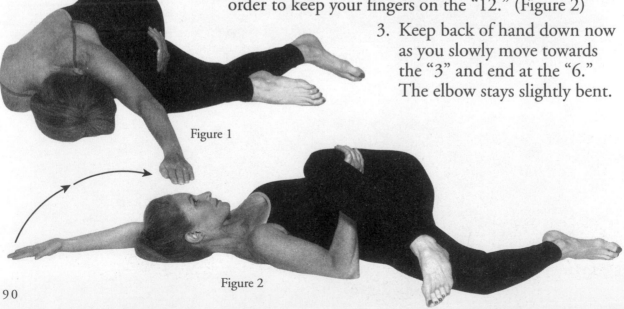

Figure 1

Figure 2

For the Hip

Position
Lie on back with both legs down, toes pointed. Arms are out to shoulder level and back of hands are on floor.

Number
Three times for each leg. Increase the intensity with each repetition.

Instructions
1. Keeping both hips and shoulders down, lift right leg one inch from the floor.
2. Keep knee slightly bent and stretch leg across body towards the number "9" on the clock. Use gravity to lengthen lower back muscles. (Figure 3)
3. Hold on behind thigh if that feels better and slowly lift leg towards the "12." Then aim for the "3" and end with the "6." (Figure 4)
4. Do three times and repeat on the other side.

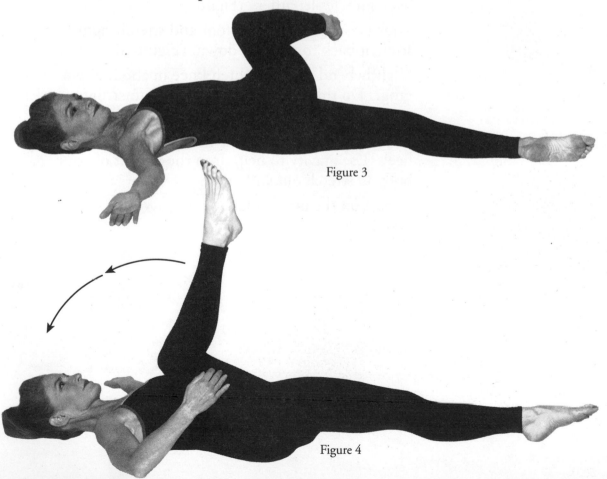

Figure 3

Figure 4

Rib/Hip Twisters

The games we played as children used to twist
and bend us as a matter of course. But so many of today's activities
are sedentary that we're not as naturally limber as before.
This exercise twists you in all directions while working as a great
spine, shoulder, hip, and ankle loosener. Keeping the
Muscle Memory Quiz in mind, think of increasing the space
between the hips and ribs as you do this exercise

Note: At first, you may feel more comfortable doing only instruction #1 and then sitting back towards the heels.

Position
Start on hands and knees.

Number
Once on each side.

Instructions

1. Stretch left arm underneath body. Lower head and left shoulder to floor. Reach beyond your fingertips and feel rib cage stretching. Keep belly pulled in and feel back muscles lengthen. (Figure 1)

2. Tuck toes under on right foot and stretch right leg straight back to pull hip down. (Figure 2)

3. Slightly bend and straighten knee in about a two-inch range. Do this five times. Feel your hamstring muscles stretching and use your leg to pull your hip down.

4. Bring left leg in, round over, and sit back towards the heels. Use gravity to help drop the weight of your body to stretch out stiff ankles.

5. Repeat on the other side.

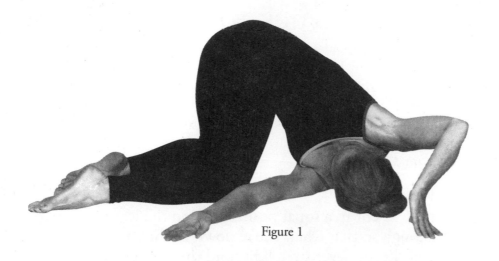

Figure 1

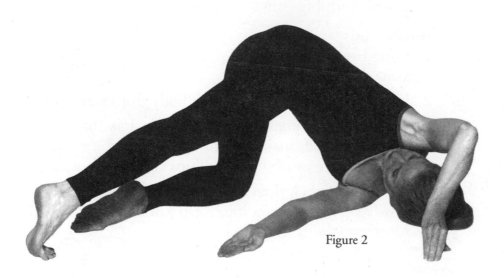

Figure 2

Squat to Stand
Tuck to Stand

I enjoy choreographing every workout so that I feel graceful
when I move. Here are two ways to make the transition from stretches
practiced lying down to those you do standing up. Use either or both as
you wish but I recommend using the Tuck to Stand if your knees hurt.
Your calf muscles always benefit from extra stretching.

Squat to Stand

Position

Knees bent in a squat position. Keep the legs wide apart,
enough so that when you're down in the squat position,
your knees never stretch beyond the middle of the top of
your feet. Turn hips out so toes are at a 45-degree angle.

Instructions

1. Drop head and shoulders down towards the floor with
   arms dangling down.

2. Lift one heel at a time and shift body from side to side.

3. Keeping abdominals pulled in tightly, raise halfway
   up. Place hands inside thighs to increase the stretch in
   your hips. Twist rib cage and hips from side to side.

4. Lift chest higher, then drop hips, and
   slowly curl up to standing. Keep knees
   soft throughout. (Figure 1)

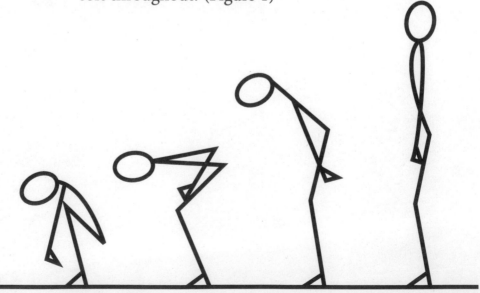

Figure 1

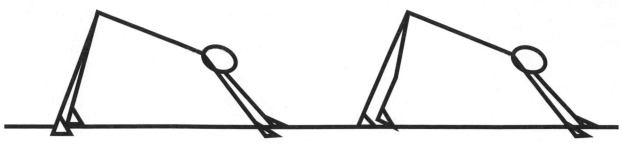

Figure 2

Tuck to Stand

Position
Begin in round-back position on hands and knees.

Instructions
1. Tuck toes under, raise tailbone, and stretch legs straight back.
2. Keep heels high as you lean body weight forward. Shift hips, lift one heel at a time, and walk feet from side to side. With abdominals pulled in, feel your back, hamstring, and calf muscles (gastrocnemius and soleus) stretching.
3. Knees slightly bent, bring hands in towards feet and slowly curl up to standing. (Figure 2)

Windmill

Open your body to experience the free feeling of a windmill.
With constant awareness of alignment, stretch all your muscles and joints
and fill your lungs with fresh air. Work slowly and smoothly and keep the
muscles balanced between your front and back.

Note: As you do instructions 1 and 2, bend lower on each repetition, pulling ribs in front down and lifting them in the back for a more intense stretch.

Position
Stand with legs spread wide apart, arms down, and align yourself.

Number
Five times, alternating each arm.

Instructions
1. Reach right arm diagonally up toward the "11" as though you were facing a clock and pull up back of rib cage. Lift right heel and press against the ball of your foot to pull up even higher. (Figure 1)

2. Looking toward left shoulder, twist spine and circle arm all the way back over and behind right shoulder. (Figure 2)

3. Looking over left shoulder, continue circling back and behind towards the opposite hip. (Figure 3)

4. Repeat with left arm reaching up diagonally.

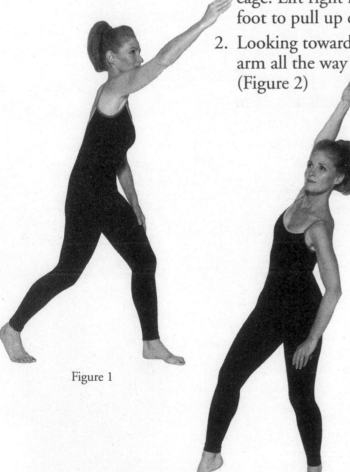

Figure 1

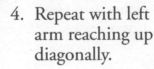

Figure 2

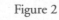

Figure 3

Opposite Elbow Bend

Whenever we use our extremities, let's remember they're connected to the core of our bodies. Because of the origin and insertion principle, moving the arm triggers movement in all the upper-back muscles and shoulder joints.

Position
Stand with legs hip-width apart and align yourself. Be sure shoulders point straight toward ceiling and are not rounded forward.

Number
Five times, alternating sides.

Instructions
1. Raise arms overhead and position them alongside ears. Keep a long space between ears and shoulders.

2. Turn left palm toward ceiling with thumb forward and place right hand on top of it. Grasp fingers together lightly. (Figure 1)

3. Bend at right elbow, keeping it close to your side, and slowly pull it all the way down. Lift left elbow as high as you can and use it to lift rib cage and define the waist. (Figure 2)

4. Stretch arms straight up and repeat on other side. Feel shoulder blades sinking in towards spine and shifting from side to side.

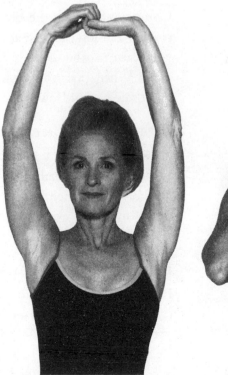

Figure 1

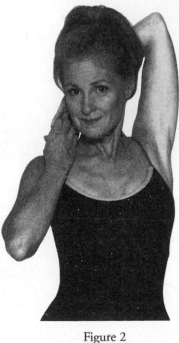

Figure 2

97

FIVE GREAT REASONS TO PRACTICE BREATHING EXERCISES

As natural as breathing is, we can do it more efficiently with practice. Breathing is both conscious and unconscious, so try to remember to pull air into your lungs as often as you can. With Muscle Memory alignment, standing up straight makes it easier to breathe well. Better breathing leads to increased lung capacity and more stamina. Exhaling properly helps you tighten your abdominals.

Breathe for Your Health

Oxygen nourishes all of the cells in the body. Each inhalation is accompanied by a deep exhalation that eliminates used air and makes room for fresh air. The lungs transfer the air we breathe in to our blood. Our hearts pump this oxygen-enriched blood to the body's tissues, including the muscles, where it combines with fuel sources and produces energy. The blood then carries waste products like carbon dioxide (CO_2) back to the lungs to release into the atmosphere.

We exercise our lungs to prevent them from becoming stiff and less elastic. The more oxygen we supply, the more efficient our bodies become at utilizing it and we become more fit.

Breathe for Relaxation

Complete focus on the breathing exercises helps free your mind of clutter. Tension causes you to breathe at a faster and less even rate. If you learn to slow down and regulate your breath, it will help you relax. When this works and you are truly relaxed, your pulse and heart rate become lower and healthier.

Breathe to Combat Stress

Stressful lives cause emotional agitation. The "fight or flight" reflex is the body's adrenaline-fueled reaction to threatening situations. This response is helpful when you need to escape a truly threatening situation. But in everyday, less serious situations, this reaction causes chemical and physical effects that damage the body.

Breathe to Increase Power

Professional athletes know they get their best performances when they're relaxed. Because a tense muscle has to be relaxed before it can perform at the highest level, relaxation becomes very important. Relaxed muscles work best. This is the same for recreational athletes. We all need to be pumped up to do our best in sports, but we need relaxation as well.

To help you relax and achieve a feeling of calmness, borrow from the Japanese method of focusing on the Hara. The Hara is at the center of your belly, about an inch lower than your navel. Start your breath at that point and concentrate on how relaxing it feels.

Breathe to Improve Your Skin

Skin is susceptible to influences from inside and outside your body. Improved breathing transports oxygenated blood to the skin's surface for a healthy, rosy glow. Tension changes the way your skin looks: Jaw clenching, forehead frowning, and mouth grimacing cause wrinkles and creases. Breathing exercises relax you and help lessen your tension.

Your face has muscles and, like all muscles, these have to be exercised and toned to look good. Feel your face muscles work with this breathing method: Inhale and tightly squeeze closed eyes and mouth. Exhale and widely open your eyes and mouth, sticking your tongue out.

In Chinese medicine, skin is referred to as the second set of lungs. Charts show how different parts of the face relate to different organs. Skin is the largest organ in the body. There is respiration through the skin. The heart, lungs, and kidneys work together to cleanse the blood. By perspiring through the skin, we eliminate carbon dioxide and other waste products.

To Begin

Breathe in the manner that feels most natural. Sit comfortably in a quiet place and practice breathing for five minutes. Close your eyes and focus on the breath moving in and out. This helps you become aware of your muscle habits. Breathe slowly and stay in a steady rhythm. Listen to the sound your breathing makes. Try doing it for ten minutes.

Whenever you need to relax, use breathing. You'll enjoy the refreshed feeling of letting go of tension.

The Method

The intercostals (between the ribs) and the diaphragm are the main muscles of respiration. The diaphragm is a large dome-shaped sheet of muscle that begins at the bottom of the sternum and inserts in the lower thorax near the belly. It separates the thoracic and abdominal cavities.

When you inhale, the diaphragm contracts, flattens, and moves downward toward the abdominal cavity. You increase the volume of air in the chest cavity. The intercostals contract and cause the ribs to rotate and lift up and away from the body.

When you exhale, the diaphragm relaxes and moves back towards the thorax. The ribs go down and the size of the chest cavity decreases. Air moves out through the respiratory tract into the atmosphere. It's important to exhale deeply to eliminate used air and make room for fresh air.

A small volume of air, called residual lung volume (RLV), always remains in the lungs. RLV is important to keep the lungs from collapsing and to allow the exchange of oxygen and carbon dioxide between the blood and lungs.

The age-related decrease in the elasticity of lung tissue tends to increase the RLV, and leave less space for new air. Inhalation and exhalation tend to decrease. Deep-breathing exercises, which reverse this trend, are necessary to maintain a high total-lung capacity.

THE THREE-MINUTE
BREATHING RELAXATION PROGRAM

Together, the following three exercises make up the Three-Minute Breathing Relaxation. You can also do them individually, whenever you need relaxation or simply desire a moment of calmness to quiet your mind. There are different ways to practice deep breathing. All of them transport more air into and out of your lungs.

Position

Choose the most comfortable and convenient position for each of these exercises. Lying down eliminates the stress of gravity, but sitting is certainly more convenient throughout the day.

Lying down: Lie on your back with your knees bent, feet flat on floor.

Sitting: Either sit on a chair with your buttocks against the back of the chair or sit cross-legged on the floor. Keep your chest slightly forward and settle into a feeling of comfort.

Breathing

Breathe in through your nose to filter the air. Breathe out through your mouth to expel the air for a forceful exhalation.

Alternate Nostril Breathing

You breathe in through one nostril at a time and after holding
the breath in with both nostrils closed, exhale out the opposite nostril.
After a few repetitions, you'll feel your forehead and entire face relax. It's
hard to believe something so simple can relax you so effectively.

Position

The traditional hand position is to use the fingers of one
hand to close each nostril. The thumb covers the right
nostril and the fourth and fifth fingers cover the left.
You bend the second and third fingers into your palm.
A simpler position, which some people prefer, is to
use the thumb and second finger.

Time/Number

Hold each "instruction" for five seconds. Increase
amount of time when you can, keeping the breaths
in an even rhythm. Repeat three to five times.

Instructions

1. Begin with your thumb blocking the right nostril and
   take in a deep breath through the left nostril.

2. At the top of the breath, use the fourth and fifth
   fingers (or the second finger) to block the left nostril
   and hold both nostrils closed.

3. Release your thumb to open the right nostril and
   exhale through it.

4. Now repeat both sides, beginning with the left
   nostril blocked, taking a deep breath through the
   right nostril.

5. Repeat. Let your body stay quiet for a while before
   you move on.

Rib Cage Breathing

I love this way of breathing because it offers another opportunity to lift the rib cage. Because your posture is affected by the downward gravitational pull, rather than sitting, do this breathing either lying down or standing. Think of blowing your lungs up like a balloon, and then letting the air out slowly.

Position
Lie on your back with your knees bent and feet flat on floor, hip-width apart. Arms are at your side.

Number
Five times.

Instructions
1. Check that lower belly is concave and neck and shoulders are relaxed.
2. Stretch arms straight up over your head as you inhale deeply through your nose. Feel entire rib cage, front and back, lifting.
3. Drop one arm down at a time as you exhale.
4. Wobble your head and shoulders to relax before each of the inhalations.

Four-Stage Abdominal Breathing

This is one of the only times I'll recommend you blow up your belly rather than keeping your abdominals from protruding. With this method, you'll experience a full range of breathing by coordinating abdominal and rib cage breathing. The goal is to move the diaphragm up and down and increase the abdominal and lung volume and capacity.

Position
Whether standing, sitting, or lying down, place hands lightly on belly. Try to connect your mental awareness to the part of your body that is moving with each instruction. Remember to keep your neck and shoulders relaxed throughout.

Number
Three to five, slowly and rhythmically.

Instructions
1. Keeping abdominals completely relaxed, inhale through your nose and fill your belly with air.

2. Continue the inhalation as you open your chest and fill your lungs with air.

3. Lungs stay full with the rib cage lifted as you exhale first from your belly. Now pull in the abdominals to increase the force of the exhalation.

4. Complete the exercise by expelling all of the air in your lungs.

5. Feel the size of the abdominal and rib cage cavities increasing and decreasing due to the position of the diaphragm.

6. Keep the front and back of your rib cage balanced and lifted. Wobble your neck and shoulders to relax.

CHAPTER FIVE

Working with Weights to Increase Bone Density and Shape Muscles

Stress! Can this be good for you? *Physical* stress in the form of intelligent exercise is a potent stimulus to maintain and increase bone mass. The bone picks up more calcium each time it is stressed. Resistance training—using weights to increase muscle strength— creates the right kind of pressure on your bones. In addition to strengthening your muscles, the Daily Ten Workout stresses your bones which adds to their strength. Every time a muscle pulls on a bone, bends it, or makes it move, bone cell growth is stimulated.

Love Your Bones

A primary health goal at any age is to build and maintain strong bones. Bone mass is the quantity of collagen, minerals, salts, and bone marrow that makes up bones. Several lifestyle factors affect our bones. Extended bed rest will reduce bone mass. But, with activity, the mass returns. At the beginning of space travel, we learned that astronauts lost bone mass in space. Even doing exercise in that environment didn't prevent the loss. That's because gravity plays an important role in maintaining bone mass. Weight-bearing exercises done against the force of gravity strengthen bones. Currently, researchers are working to develop exercise equipment to become part of the spacecraft. Through simulating the earth's mechanical stress on the bones in the presence of gravity, these machines would help prevent bone loss.

Throughout life, your bones undergo a continuous process of reconstruction and reshaping. Worn out bone is automatically replaced by new bone. This active remodeling process takes place until approximately age twenty. Growth continues until about age thirty, and then peak bone mass is reached. Beyond that, remodeling processes go on, but at a much slower pace.

Regardless of age, people who maintain an active lifestyle have significantly greater bone mass than sedentary people. Bones get stronger at the specific sites where the muscles are pulling, because a "peizoelectric crystal" forms. This crystal transforms mechanical stress from a physical activity into electrical energy which stimulates bone-forming cells at the point of the stress. This is why a professional tennis player's dominant arm has a thicker bone mass than the other. Keep this in mind when you exercise with weights. Continued physical force on your skeleton remodels the bones. Make bone-building a lifelong commitment. In the absence of an ongoing program, bone mass reverts back to its pre-exercise levels.

Osteoporosis is a disease characterized by the loss of bone mass. Bones become fragile and are vulnerable to fractures. One half of all fractures due to osteoporosis occur in the vertebrae in the upper spine. When these bones become thin and weak, they can't support your head and neck or keep your spine straight. This condition is preventable. Although it is possible to develop a "dowager's hump" and actually become shorter, you can regain lost height by learning how to straighten your spine. Keep the rest of the body in alignment with Muscle Memory. These strategies help you fight osteoporosis.

Shape Your Muscles as You Save Your Bones

Strengthening exercises also increase the number and size of muscle fibers. Each muscle fiber will have more power to give you better endurance and less fatigue. Muscle strength is the force your muscle can exert against resistance. Endurance is the ability of your muscle to exert force over a long period of time. Having strength and endurance adds to your physicality and your ability to remain active. You won't have to work as hard to accomplish strenuous tasks once you've increased your strength and endurance.

Muscle tissue is metabolically active. Fat has little metabolic activity. Having more muscles changes your body composition and helps you look lean and fit. Use the strength training exercises to develop and shape your muscles and the Intelligent Walking Program in Chapter Six to decreases your percentage of body fat. Drastically restricting your caloric intake means your fat loss will usually be accompanied by loss of lean weight or muscle. This will lower your metabolic rate. Then you'll have to exercise harder and restrict your calories even further to lose weight.

Basic Strength

How much strength do you need to manage every day? This is a basic program. It isn't about becoming a body builder. The Arm Exercises will help maintain strength and prevent your upper arms from sagging. Arm strength is an advantage in sports and in just about everything else. The thoracic vertebrae in your upper and middle back will be strengthened by the arm exercises and this prevents your spine from curving.

The Standing Hip and Thigh Strengthener works your largest muscles. You need strong legs to anchor yourself in many activities, whether for your golf swing or climbing up stairs.

Muscles and bones get their training effects in the same way. Increases in specific sites result from exercises that are localized for those sites. In the standing exercise, the thigh bone and lumbar spine (lower back) receive extra bone-building stress because you have to work all these muscles to stay upright against the downward gravitational pull.

Following the Arm Exercises and the Standing Hip and Thigh Strengthener, you'll find Wrist Strengtheners and Ankle Strengtheners. We use these areas a lot and sometimes we overuse and strain them. They need to be strong to prevent injuries. Even turning a doorknob can become painful if your wrists are weak. When I had my bone density measured at age forty-eight, the results from my hips and spine showed a bone mass that was equivalent to that of a much younger woman. Given my career as a fitness expert and my healthy lifestyle, I wouldn't have expected otherwise. However, I was surprised that the bone density in my wrist corresponded to that of a forty-eight-year old. This reinforced the concept that we must do exercises specific to every site in the body. So I began these wrist exercises and now that I'm fifty, my wrists are younger.

Try to support your entire exercise program with a healthy eating plan so you don't deprive your bones of necessary nutrients. It is very important to ingest and absorb calcium at every age. Your bone-building cells—called osteoblasts—need calcium to do their work. Calcium also regulates muscle contractions. Milk, of course, has calcium. Are you aware of which food habits deplete calcium? When taken in excess, sugar, caffeine, phosphates (in soft drinks), and alcohol can draw calcium out of your body. It's a good idea to ask your physician how you can meet your calcium requirements.

Before You Begin

Every aspect of Muscle Memory comes into play when you're doing weight-bearing exercises. By staying straight and tall from your feet up through your head, you'll harness all your strength and feel balanced and centered.

The origin and insertion principle ensures that you're getting an optimal result from each movement. For example, the origin of the triceps is along the upper arm and underneath the shoulder blade. Balance the chest and upper-back muscles and keep your shoulder pointed straight up when you exercise your triceps. If your shoulders hunch forward, the upper back gets rounded and you lose the position needed to stablize the triceps.

Weights

These exercises can be done with or without weights, although I think they are more effective with them. Begin without dumbbells and imagine you're holding a heavy weight and can overcome the resistance of that weight to move. Using weights such as dumbbells makes the arm feel heavier and increases the difficulty of each exercise. But regardless of the size of the weight and even if you have no weight, imagine that it has a "will of its own" that your muscle has to overcome. Even a one-pound weight can have a determined will not to be lifted or lowered. Start the motion from the muscle, not from the weight.

The simplest way to train for increased strength is to use your own body weight. One of the Daily Ten, the Positive Push-up, strengthens your arms, shoulders, and chest. Instead of holding a weight, your body becomes the weight that your arms have to lift and lower. Walking strengthens your legs. By adding this Strength Training, you're going a step beyond and working towards additional strength, bone density, and muscle shaping.

When you feel comfortable, invest in an inexpensive pair of dumbbells. They allow freedom of movement, unlike most machines and weight bars. This lessens the stress to your joints. When you select a pair of dumbbells, you'll want them to have enough resistance to tire the working muscle within eight to twelve repetitions first in one and then in two sets. Over-training with weights that are too heavy will lead to injury. Try out one-, two-, or three-pound weights in the store. Ask the sales person to gauge your strength and help you select the correct weight.

Dumbbell Smarts

After working out with dumbbells for the first time, evaluate how you feel the following day. If you are sore, do fewer repetitions or do not use weights the next time you exercise. Leave at least one day in between your weight-training workouts.

If your shoulders feel irritated, don't work out with dumbbells. Keep the shoulders moving and try the Arm Exercises without weights. Only when your shoulders feel comfortable—without pain—should you re-introduce the weights.

Always keep circulation in a joint and stop whatever causes pain. "Active rest" is what I call the healing process.

When exercising with weights, any body segment that is out of line will have to strain and work harder to maintain itself and prevent injury. If you're holding weights straight up to the ceiling and your neck and shoulders are hunched, they'll hunch and strain even more under a heavy weight. If you're leaning your torso back, your belly will stick out and your back will tense. Having practiced and achieved that lovely look of alignment through your Daily Ten and Muscle Memory, put it to work for you in your strengthening exercises.

Back Benefits

The muscle name listed in each exercise is the *primary* muscle you'll be working. You'll feel additional muscles working with the primary muscle automatically, but keep your focus on the primary muscle.

Ballet dancers have very strong arms and upper backs. Every time they have to hold up their arms to keep a pose—often for several moments—they are automatically strengthening their backs. In all of your arm exercises, like a ballerina, you'll strengthen the muscles of your upper back, including the latissimus, rhomboids, and trapezius.

Muscle Memory Review

Emphasize proper form to reinforce your Muscle Memory motor-learning process and stay focused. Know where the primary working muscle is, its origin, and insertion.

Try to use as many of the Muscle Memory Quiz questions as you can. For example, the trapezius muscle, which originates in your back and inserts at the base of your skull, can cause your shoulders to hunch while doing arm exercises. Here's where the first three Muscle Memory Quiz questions apply:

- Is there a long space between my ear and shoulder?

Extra Help

- Never lock a joint or hyperextend it. For example, in the biceps and triceps exercises, the elbow must stay relaxed because both muscles insert at that point. Same for the shoulder, the wrist, hips, knees, and ankles: they all stay relaxed.
- Be sure you're not using too heavy a weight as this adds too much stress to the joint.
- Work against gravity. Give it an imaginary form. Use your muscles to counteract it.
- Keep your arm movements smooth and steady. Work slowly enough to isolate the muscles. Don't rely on momentum.
- Involve your whole body. Even when you're doing arm exercises, your legs form a strong base and stabilize the body. Abdominals stabilize the ribs and pelvis.

- Is the back of my head in the same line as my upper back?
- Do my shoulders point straight to the ceiling?

YOUR PROGRAM

A **repetition** or **rep** is one complete movement of the exercise. A **set** is a given number of repetitions of the specific exercise that are done consecutively without a rest. A **rest** is the pause in between sets. **Resistance** is the heaviness of the dumbbell.
- Two to three days per week.
- One to two sets of eight to twelve repetitions per exercise.
- Be sure your muscle feels fatigued at the end of the set.
  If not, use a heavier weight.

Breathing

Breathing helps avoid stress during weight training. Inhale through your nose to begin the exercise. Exhale through your mouth on the maximum effort. Think of directing the breath to the belly of your working muscle. Squeeze in hard at that point and "set" it. You can't really blow the breath all the way there, but this technique helps you focus and feel the work in the belly of the muscle. Inhale through your nose as you return to the starting position.

Number

Try each exercise without dumbbells and review your Muscle Memory. Next, do two or three passive repetitions with dumbbells to warm up the muscle. Now you're ready to increase the intensity.

When you keep your concentration and intensity high, one set of eight repetitions may be sufficient. Some weight-lifting techniques recommend light weights with more repetitions, others use heavy weights and fewer repetitions. If, after a while, you find the exercise feels too easy, add a second or third set. You may try a heavier weight, but remember to keep the exercise comfortable and your form correct. Most of my students work up to three-pound dumbbells and a few use five-pound dumbbells.

One More Word

To put your body in alignment before you begin your strength training, do the One-Minute Muscle Memory Boost.

Triceps One

Along the Back of Upper Arm

Position
Stand with legs shoulder-width apart, arms down at sides. Keep knees unlocked.

Instructions
1. Roll shoulders back and down, keeping shoulder blades in.

2. Stretch arms back at an angle. Try to keep shoulder pointed toward ceiling. Do not allow it to roll forward.

3. Lift and bend elbows. Keep upper arms alongside body.

4. Slowly straighten arms back, tensing triceps. Hold and "set." (Figure 1)

5. Bend arms and repeat, keeping upper arms still, elbows high, and shoulders down.

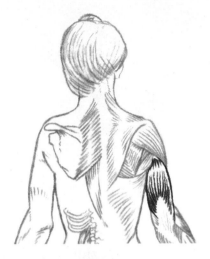

Primary Muscle Used:

Triceps

Origin: Shoulder blade *(scapula)* and upper arm *(humerus)*
Insertion: Elbow bone *(ulna)*

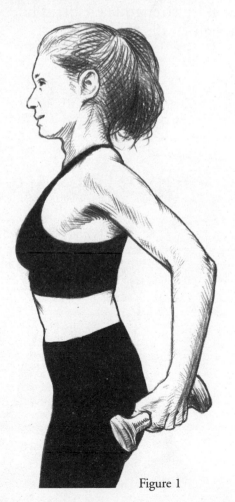

Figure 1

Your Muscle Memory Voice
➤ *Is the back of my head in the same line as my upper back?*
➤ *Is my chest more forward than my belly?*

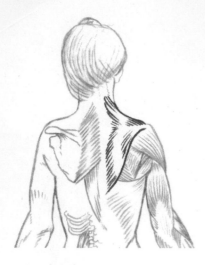

Trapezius

Across Upper Back and Back of Neck

Position

Stand with legs about three feet apart with knees and toes pointed out at a 45-degree angle. Knees are slightly bent, pointing in the same direction as feet.

Instructions

1. Arms down in front with a dumbbell in each hand, palms facing your thighs.

2. Keeping shoulders down, lift and bend elbows up and back.

3. With elbows and hands higher than shoulders, pull shoulder blades together and feel the spine in the upper back sinking in. (Figure 1)

4. Slowly lower arms down and repeat.

5. Optional leg strengthener: Bend knees 3 inches on #1 and straighten on #2.

Primary Muscle Used:

Trapezius

Origin: Spine of middle back *(thoracic spine)* and back of neck *(cervical spine)*
Insertion: Collar bone *(clavicle),* top of shoulder blade *(scapula),* and base of skull *(cervical spine)*

Your Muscle Memory Voice

➤ *Is there a long space between my ear and shoulder?*
➤ *Do my shoulders point straight to the ceiling?*
➤ *Do I feel the same strength in my chest and upper back?*

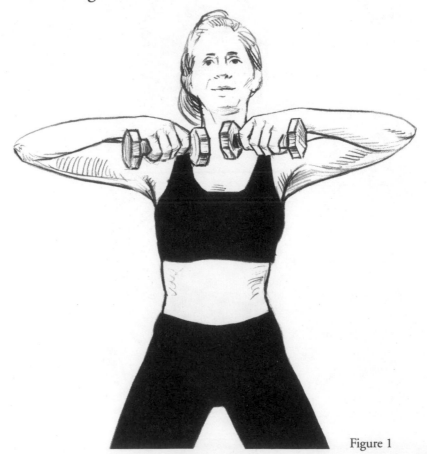

Figure 1

Deltoids

At Top of Shoulders

Position
Stand with legs shoulder-width apart.

Instructions
1. With palm facing down, squeeze at the shoulder and slowly raise left arm straight in front to shoulder height. (1 set.)
2. Slowly lower and repeat with right arm. (1 set.)
3. Raise and lower both arms at the same time. (2 sets.) (Figure 1)

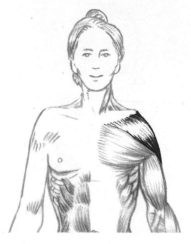

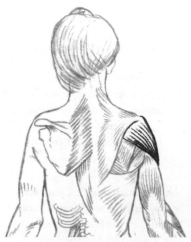

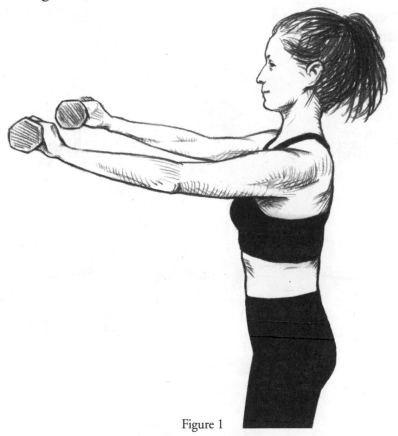

Figure 1

Primary Muscle Used:

Deltoids

Origin: Collarbone (back of *clavicle)* and shoulder blade (top of *scapula)*
Insertion: Upper arm bone (middle of *humerus)*

Your Muscle Memory Voice
➤ *Is the back of my head in the same line as my upper back?*
➤ *Is there a long space between my ear and shoulder?*

ALTERNATIVE EXERCISE:
Position
Stand with legs shoulder-width apart.
Instructions
1. With palms facing in, slowly raise arms sideways up to shoulder height.
2. Slowly lower and repeat.

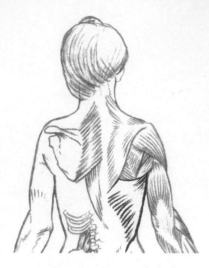

Latissimus Dorsi
Across Back of Ribs

Primary Muscle Used:
Latissimus Dorsi

Origin: Middle back
(thoracic vertebrae), lower back
(lumbar and *sacral vertebrae)*,
top of pelvis
Insertion: Shoulder (top of
humerus)

Note: Touch and feel your **latissimus muscle** working. It's usually unfamilar because you only see it when looking at your back in a mirror. Most of us are stronger in our arms and shoulders and use those muscles too much during this exercise. Keep the latissimus the focus of the movement.

Your Muscle Memory Voice
➤ *Is the back of my head in the same line as my upper back?*
➤ *Do I feel the same strength in my chest and upper back?*
➤ *Am I pulling my ribs in front down and lifting the ribs in back?*

Position
Stand with legs shoulder-width apart.

Instructions
1. Bend arms at a right angle. Lift elbows to the same height as shoulders.
2. Straighten arms toward ceiling. Keep wrist, elbow, and shoulder in a straight line.
3. Using latissimus across back of ribs, bend elbows and pull arms down to a right angle. (Figure 1)
4. Feel the mid-back (thoracic spine) pulling in. "Set" and repeat.

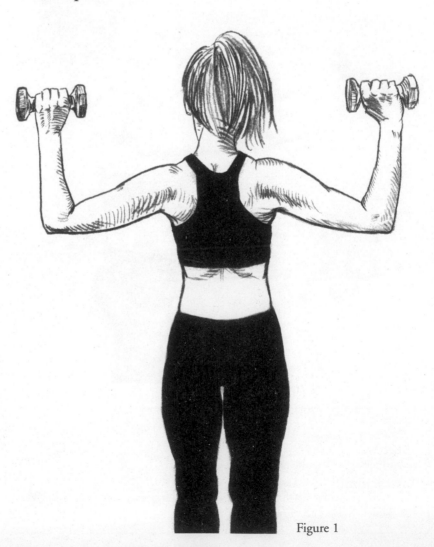

Figure 1

114

Triceps Two

Along the Back of Upper Arm

As I'll explain more fully in Chapter Six, muscle
tissue and fat cells are different from each other and one does not
turn into the other. At the tricep muscle, a woman accumulates
a large portion of her total fat percentage. If we can increase muscle
fiber at that site, we'll burn away fat more successfully.

This variation for strengthening triceps offers a slightly different effect.
If we make twice the effort, we'll get twice the benefits!

Position
Stand with legs shoulder-width apart.

Instructions
1. Begin with arms straight up toward ceiling, alongside ear.
2. Bend arms, keeping elbows high and upper arms still. (Figure 1)
3. Squeezing the triceps, slowly straighten arms. Hold and "set."
4. Bend arms and repeat.

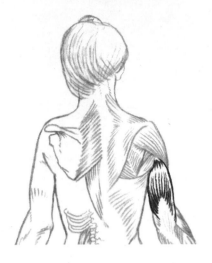

Primary Muscle Used:

Triceps

Origin: Shoulder blade *(scapula)*
and upper arm *(humerus)*
Insertion: Elbow bone *(ulna)*

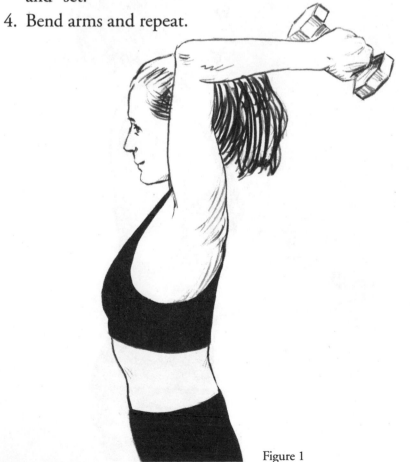

Figure 1

Your Muscle Memory Voice
➤ *Is there a long space between my ear and shoulder?*
➤ *Do I feel the same strength in my chest and upper back?*
➤ *Is my chest more forward than my belly?*

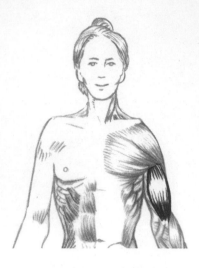

Biceps
Front of Upper Arm

Position
Stand with legs shoulder-width apart.

Instructions
1. Begin with arms down, palms facing forward.
2. Bend one arm and curl dumbbell towards shoulder, stopping halfway up.
3. Tense biceps, hold, and "set."
4. Keeping elbows still, hold the tension as you straighten back down and repeat.

Primary Muscle Used:

Biceps

Origin: Upper arm bone *(humerus),* outer edge of shoulder blade *(scapula)*
Insertion: Elbow bone (top of *radius)*

Note: Because we use the biceps as part of ordinary movements, it is stronger than its partner, the triceps. When you feel ready, increase the weight you're lifting by holding two dumbbells in the working hand as you work each arm individually.

Your Muscle Memory Voice
➤ *Do my shoulders point straight to the ceiling?*
➤ *Are my leg muscles balanced so my knee is aligned and not stiff?*

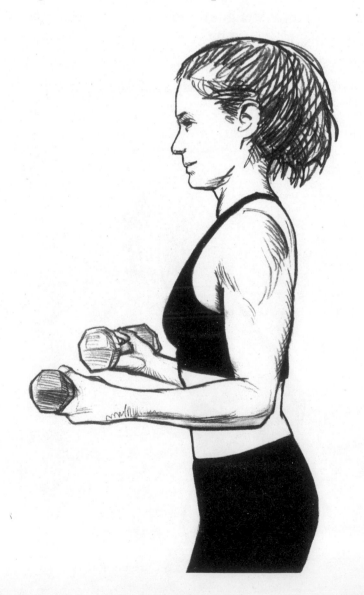

Recovery Stretch for Arm Strengtheners

1. Stretch one arm across chest. Hold on to that elbow with the other hand.

2. Gently pull on the elbow until you feel a pleasing stretch in the shoulder. Breathe naturally and hold for a count of 10.

3. Be sure you're not scrunching up your shoulder and that you keep a long space between your ear and shoulder.

4. Repeat on the other side.

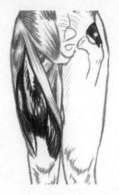

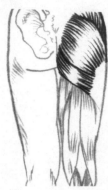

Primary Muscles Used:

Gluteus and Quadriceps

Muscle: Gluteus
Origin: Hip *(ilium)*, tailbone *(sacrum)*
Insertion: Top of thigh bone *(femur)*

Muscle: Quadriceps
Origin: Hip *(ilium)*, top of thighbone *(femur)*
Insertion: Just below knee cap *(patella)*

Standing Hip and Thigh Strengtheners

When you exercise for a specific area, the muscles and bones in that area get stronger. This isn't spot reducing, which really doesn't work. This is spot toning, whereby you increase the number and size of muscle fibers. Your leg and buttocks muscles are the largest in the body and they respond well to exercise.

Number

One set of 12 repetitions; work up to 25 repetitions.

Position

Stand with legs about three feet apart with knees and toes pointed out at a 45-degree angle. Keep knees pointing in same direction as feet.

Instructions

1. Hold dumbbells down in front of you.

2. Slowly lower body, stopping when thighs are almost parallel to floor and knees are over the middle of feet. Never press knees beyond toes.

3. With a little range of motion, about 3 to 4 inches, "pulse" slowly up and down. Do not use momentum. Use your muscles to make the movement. Squeeze outer thigh muscles to move you down. Lean towards your heels. Squeeze buttocks and inner thigh muscles to move you up. (Figure 1)

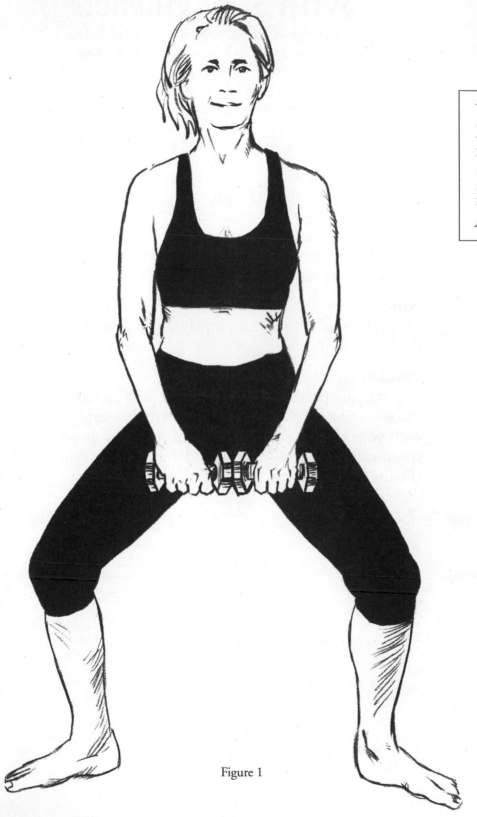

Figure 1

Your Muscle
Memory Voice
➢ *Is the back of my head in the same line as my upper back?*
➢ *Is my chest more forward than my belly?*

Wrist Strengtheners

As small as they may seem, your wrists bend up and down,
move from side to side, rotate, and circle. Wrist muscles have to be strong
and flexible just like all the other muscles in your body. You
have flexor and extensor wrist muscles which have to be balanced. The
wrist is delicate. These exercises will help you avoid overuse injuries
that can result if your wrists are weak and you do a lot of repetitive hand
motions such as working on a computer.

Before You Begin
Bend your arms at a right angle and stand with your
elbows close to your waist. Exercise for one week without
holding dumbbells, then use a one-pound weight in each
hand. Build up to three-pound weights only when you
can do the exercise without any strain.

Number
Do each exercise five times slowly and repeat every other
day.

Position
The starting position for each of the four exercises is with
the wrist and fingers flat, palms down, in a straight line
with your shoulder and elbow. Use the wrist muscles
specifically and keep your shoulder and upper arm still.
(Figure 1)

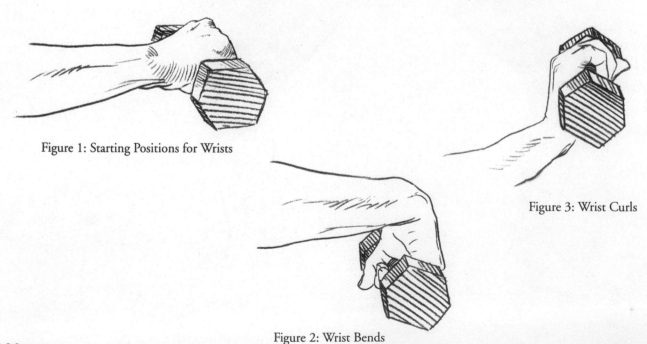

Figure 1: Starting Positions for Wrists

Figure 3: Wrist Curls

Figure 2: Wrist Bends

Wrist Bends

1. Bend your wrist down and "set" for five seconds. (Figure 2)

2. Return to starting position.

Wrist Curls

1. Flex your wrists up and "set" for five seconds. (Figure 3)

2. Return to starting position.

Wrist Windshield Wipers

1. Keep your wrists on the same plane and move them from side to side like windshield wipers. Keep your forearms still. (Figure 4)

Wrist Rotators

1. Begin with your wrists and forearms facing down, parallel to the floor.

2. Turn your wrists and forearms so they face up, parallel to the ceiling, and "set" for five seconds. (Figure 5)

3. Turn your wrists and forearms back to the starting position.

Recovery Stretch

1. Make five slow wrists circles in both directions.

> ## Your Muscle Memory Voice
> ➤ *Is there a long space between my ear and shoulder?*
> ➤ *Can I drop a plumb line from the ceiling and have it go down the center of each body segment in a straight line?*

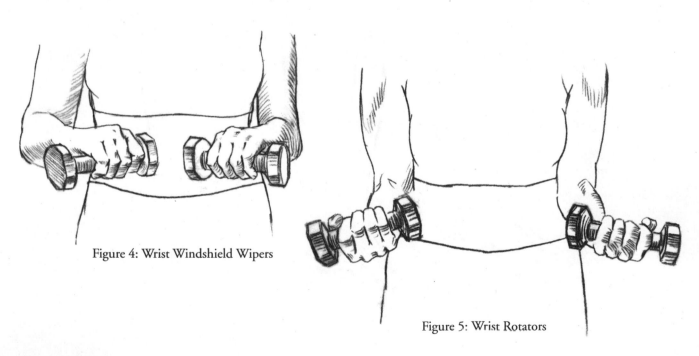

Figure 4: Wrist Windshield Wipers

Figure 5: Wrist Rotators

Foot and Ankle Strengtheners

As good as the rest of your body feels, your mood can drop
if your feet hurt. And after they're cooped up all day inside shoes, it's
a treat for them to be stretched and strengthened. These exercises
improve circulation in the feet, strengthen the arches, and help
relieve any pressure. If your ankles feel weak, practice walking down
one flight of stairs backwards. Your ankles will get stronger.

Starting Position

It is the same for the three exercises. Sit forward on a
chair or on the side of a bed. Lift legs slightly in front.
Keep hip, knee, and foot in a straight line throughout
exercise. Be sure not to turn in your knee.

Ankle Strengthener

1. Stretch heels away, flex feet, and bring toes straight up.

2. In five counts, press down, one section of the foot at a
   time, starting with foot flexed and toes curled:

   • press heel forward (toes spread and up)

   • press down arch (toes up) (Figure 1)

   • press down ball of foot (toes up)

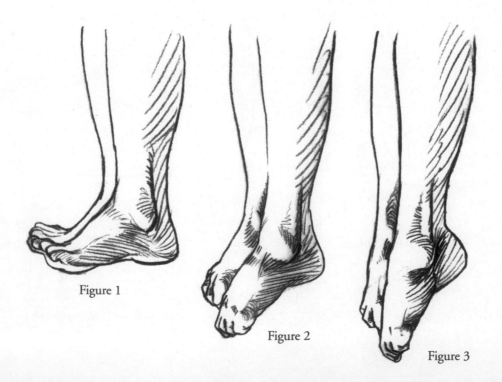

Figure 1

Figure 2

Figure 3

- press down top of foot (space on top of foot fills out) (Figure 2)
- point toes down (stretch beyond the toes) (Figure 3)

3. Curl toes and slowly return to starting position.

Practice this pattern with your hands and feel how complete the stretch is. Your wrist moves in many directions, but your ankle only moves up and down.

Arch Strengthener A

1. Press feet down and point toes.

2. Keep heels still as you bring big toes together to form an upside down letter "V." (Figure 4)

3. Feel arches pulling up, hold, and "set" for five seconds.

4. Relax and let go.

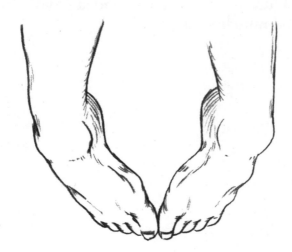

Figure 4

Arch Strengthener B

1. Stretch heels away, flex feet, and curl toes.

2. Keep heels still as you bring big toes together to form an upside down letter "V." (Figure 4) Keep big toe and pinky toe even as though they both are touching a piece of paper.

3. Repeat Steps 3 and 4 above.

Recovery Stretch

1. Foot circles: Turn in toes, press ankles down, and prescribe circles with feet.

Standing Relax And Stretch

Position
Stand with legs hip-width apart.

Instructions

1. Drop head and shoulders and hang over.

2. Keep knees slightly bent and curl up only 3 inches. Feel back and hamstring muscles stretching.

3. Drop back down and use the additional weight of the dumbbells to increase your stretch.

4. Repeat four times, then put the dumbbells down, and roll up slowly to a standing position.

Roll back your shoulders and answer all ten Muscle Memory Quiz questions. You've added to your bone density and muscle strength!

CHAPTER SIX

Intelligent Walking for Cardio Fitness and Weight Management

Now take your Muscle Memory Voice for a walk. The world's easiest and most accessible physical activity—walking—provides basic aerobic fitness. If you are new to exercise, walking is the best way to experience the deep breathing, total exhilaration, and almost instant health benefits of an aerobic workout. If you are already a committed walker or jogger or use an indoor exercise machine, applying Muscle Memory will enhance your workout.

Many activities can increase your cardiovascular fitness. Do you play tennis? Swim? Hike? Dance? Ride a bike? These and other sports give you additional conditioning but they are "stop and go" activities. They don't keep you at a constant target heart rate. Play and engage in recreational sports for the fun and physicality. But to achieve a meaningful level of cardiovascular fitness and to manage your weight, you need a more sustained aerobic workout.

As important as the Daily Ten workout is for establishing Muscle Memory…as vital as the Stretch and Joint Loosener is to increase flexibility and prevent stiffness…as beneficial as Working with Weights is to shape muscles and build bone density…your fitness cannot be considered complete without the aerobic component.

Starting a walking program is easy. Just walking briskly, slightly uphill, for thirty minutes a day is great. For more substantial results, include some hills that make you work harder. Turn your walk into an intelligent and efficient aerobic activity by applying Muscle Memory principles and by working toward your target heart rate.

Walk for Your Health

The medical benefits of walking are miraculous. Walking will enrich your lifestyle and create a higher level of endurance and health.

Energy production in the body depends on the utilization of oxygen. Lung capacity will increase as you exercise aerobically. Your goal is to keep the muscles conditioned and efficient at using oxygen so that you have correct energy transfer and your heart does not have to work overtime. VO_2 MAX is the ability of the body to take in oxygen and transport it for use in the oxidation of fuel. It is one formula we use to measure our maximum aerobic power. "V" is for volume and "O_2" stands for oxygen. With this ability, you can do strenuous activity without becoming breathless. After age twenty-five, the maximum VO_2 declines at about 1 percent per year. Doing sustained aerobic exercise comfortably will maintain your VO_2 MAX.

A regular walking program can help lower your blood pressure and increase your circulation. Muscles get food and oxygen from the blood. Walking will improve the health of your heart by raising the "good" HDL cholesterol and lowering the "bad" LDL cholesterol, which clogs your arteries.

Walking helps keep your body lean and strong. It emphasizes the lower body muscles, the ones whose shape we would all like to improve. Strong leg muscles are essential to a lifelong ability to climb stairs without getting winded, get out of cars gracefully, and stride down the street confidently.

Walking not only increases muscle strength, your bones get stronger, too. As I told you in Chapter Five, this is due to the action of the "peizoelectric crystal," which uses the mechanical stress of exercise to stimulate bone growth. Every time a muscle pulls on a bone, the extra pressure helps maintain its density. To build bone, you must exert energy against the force of gravity. Significant muscular force is generated against the long skeletal bones with every step. Measurable increases in bone mass can result. With walking, you have controlled impact. This strengthens your bones without putting excessive pressure on your joints. Walking up and down stairs strengthens muscles and adds bone. Because walking *up* stairs seems more strenuous, you might think it is more beneficial than walking down. Yes, climbing the stairs strengthens the muscles. But, in addition, when walking *down* stairs, muscles pull on bones to resist gravity. More bone-building benefits result.

All women can help reduce the future risk of bone loss and the potential for fractures with a walking program.

Joints need to stay flexible and our skeletons need to stay strong. The "itis" endings start creeping into our vocabulary as we get older. Thus our health goals will change. We want to know how to prevent not only the bone loss associated with osteoporosis but to alleviate the symptoms of osteoarthritis, tendonitis, and bursitis as well.

Walking is excellent for weight management. Your metabolism and fat-burning capacity increase and you can move away from the dieting mentality. Consistent aerobic exercise leads not only to weight loss but also to a reduction in body fat percentage. This fights the predictable muscle loss and fat gain that usually accompany getting older.

So walk! Walk to work. Walk to do errands. Use stairs whenever you can. Let your legs be your preferred mode of transportation.

Walk for Tranquillity

Walking makes you feel better and helps reduce stress. Because it uses only part of your total physical capacity, it doesn't fatigue you as much as other activities. Your core body temperature rises and a pleasurable warmth spreads into all your pores. You are always rewarded for whatever effort you made to take your walk. Mood-lifting endorphins create a mildly euphoric mental state that calms you down and clears away tension. When you don't get to take a walk, you'll find you really miss it.

Walking can be meditative. Your mind quiets as you become aware of your breathing. It can provide you with private time to think or to empty your mind of daily worries.

Walk with a companion. Walk to see the sights in your own town or a new city. Walking can create many opportunities for new experiences. You'll find that other people in your neighborhood are already out there in their fitness quest.

Most people feel better becoming more physical. A proud feeling comes from doing something healthy. It makes you an active participant in your health care and that's empowering.

Walk More Effectively

Alignment is vital to your walk. Picture the motion of a train—how smoothly the wheels spin. You'll learn to mirror that balanced motion. When you walk, your knee functions as a "transfer" joint between the hip and ankle. Keeping your knee in a straight line with your ankle and hip gives you smooth motion. This will protect your body from injury.

Use your back leg and push off with your back foot to propel you forward when you walk. At that moment, do not lock the back of the knee. Women tend to be more aware of the fronts of the body than the backs. We have the habit of checking whether we're holding in our stomachs, whether our bra straps are pulled up, and how our faces and hair look from the front. When we walk, we need to counteract our natural tendency to only use our quadriceps in the front rather than also using the hamstring in the back. Use the Leg Shake Recovery Stretch while standing up (keeping your feet on the ground, of course) to activate the hamstrings. Once you know how it feels to use the hamstrings, practice walking using this new awareness.

Walk for Weight Management

Government guidelines used to make weight-gain allowances for people as they aged, based on lower metabolic rates and the decline in physical activity. Today's guidelines recommend that adults stay within a single, healthy weight range throughout their lives. Fortunately, we now know how: by *raising* our metabolic rates through *increased* physical activity.

One reason women get fatter as they age is that their metabolism decreases and they burn fewer calories. Unless they decrease their caloric intake at the same rate, they're going to gain weight. As I said in Chapter One, it's typical for sedentary people after the age of twenty-five to lose a half pound of lean body weight (mainly muscle) and gain a half pound of fat each year. You can gain thirty pounds of extra fat after the age of twenty-five if you don't change some of your habits.

New statistics show that Americans are fatter now than a decade ago. Fatness is measured using a *Body Mass Index* scale. The recommended Body Mass Index is under 25. Here's how to measure your BMI:

BMI = Weight in kilograms (1 lb. = .45 kg.)
Divided by height in meters squared
(1 meter = 39.37 inches)

Aerobic exercise raises your basal metabolism rate (BMR), and sustains this elevation for several hours after your workout. BMR is the rate of calories burned throughout an average day based on height, weight, and normal activity. This is the amount of calories you need to maintain your weight and your normal body processes, such as breathing and heartbeat. The more activity in your day, the more you increase your BMR. That's why active people can eat more, without gaining weight, than sedentary people.

There are a variety of methods for measuring your BMR. Even though my preferred method seems complex, it's a good idea to use it because it is so specific.

THE HARRIS-BENEDICT EQUATION FOR WOMEN

655 + 4.4 × weight in lbs. + 4.3 × height in inches
- 4.7 × age in years = BMR in kilocalories

A simpler way to measure your BMR follows.

HOW TO FIGURE YOUR BMR

1. Multiply your weight by 10.
2. Multiply that number by 30%. This is an estimate of the calories used in "normal" activity.
3. Add #1 and #2.

Expending more calories through physical activity will increase your BMR.

Drastically dieting does not work for long-term weight management. You lose fat when you restrict your calories, but you also lose lean weight, or muscle. This causes your BMR to drop because the body believes it is in the hibernation state and burns fewer calories. Too little food causes the body to believe it is starving. It therefore wants to conserve fuel rather than burn it.

Aerobic exercise is the most efficient way to raise your metabolism, reduce body fat, and keep it off. When you engage in an ongoing aerobic activity like walking, you expend more calories and tip the balance in your favor by creating a "negative" energy balance. You use more calories than you take in and you lose weight.

To lose one pound of fat, you have to burn 3500 calories more than you consume, since one pound of fat equals 3500 calories. A calorie is a measurement that shows the heat or energy value of food and of physical activity. It is the unit of heat necessary to raise the temperature of water one degree. If you can boost your metabolism and use 500 calories more per day by walking and being more physical in your life, you can lose one pound of fat each week.

The best approach to permanent weight loss combines consistent aerobic exercise with good nutrition and a mild caloric restriction. People who exercise aerobically several times a week have an easier time controlling their appetites and are often motivated to eat a more nutritious diet.

A realistic weight loss is 1 to 2 pounds per week. But don't let the scale be your only measure. Remember that you are building muscle with the Muscle Memory Workout and with your strength training exercises. Muscle weighs more than fat. That's why I prefer that you gauge your weight loss by how you fit into a pair of jeans that have become too tight. Two pounds of weight loss equals a loss of 1 percent body fat. Even that small a loss will make your jeans fit better. Remember, too, that my entire approach to fitness is about a long term commitment, not a quick fix. So please have the patience to give your new health and fitness program three weeks to show results. You show a greater loss in the beginning because your cells are losing water. But once you jump-start your metabolism, weight loss will continue steadily.

Decrease Fat Cells, Increase Muscle Tissue

The Muscle Memory Method is designed to create more muscle fiber. Walking builds muscle fiber at the same time that it burns fat and conditions your cardiovascular system. With more muscle you burn more fat. Extra fat is stored in fat cells, but your muscles burn fat and use it for energy. Therefore the more muscle you have, the more calories you burn.

When we are younger, we have a greater reserve of muscle and strength than we need to maintain daily activities. As we get older, let's not replace youthful muscle with fat by not exercising. Be aware that fat cells and muscle cells are different and one does not turn into the other. You cannot eliminate fat cells, but you can shrink them. The increased circulation from exercise helps remove fatty acids from adipose (fat) tissue. At the same time, as you exercise you can thicken and increase the number of muscle fibers, which increases your metabolism. Muscles respond to fat cell shrinkage by increasing the sites where fat can be burned.

Muscle is metabolically active tissue. FFB refers to the fat-free portion of your body: muscle, bone, internal organs. If you maintain a low fat percentage and high FFB as you age, you will maintain your high metabolism and look a lot more fit.

Muscle Memory and Your Walking Technique

Walking with the proper technique increases your stamina and helps prevent strains and injuries. The questions and answers in the Muscle Memory Quiz will enhance your walking technique. When you know how to control your body, whatever you do feels more comfortable. Because walking is so natural to the body, it's a very graceful activity.

Let's start our alignment checklist with the head. Keep your chin parallel to the ground, eyes straight ahead and head moved back. Some people walk with their heads and chins tucked down which results in slouching and rounded shoulders. This causes the rib cage to sink down because all your muscles lead in to one another. Your goal is to use all of your muscles to stand straight and tall, regardless of the activity.

Here's how to apply the Muscle Memory Quiz questions and answers as you walk. This may seem a little awkward at first but once your body "gets it," your walk will be greatly enhanced.

> Question 1: *Are there two long spaces in my body: Between my ear and shoulder? Between my ribs and hips?*
> Question 2: *Is the back of my head in the same line as my upper back?*

Keep your shoulders pulled back and down. This lets the pectoral muscles on your chest spread out like a fan so your chest opens and allows the lungs to take in deep breaths and exhale forcefully.

As with all exercise, remember to breathe in and out consciously. If you get a stitch in your side, you may not be breathing in deeply enough and not exhaling the used air from your lungs to make room for fresh air. Or you may be walking too fast and not delivering enough oxygen to your muscles.

When I walk, I breathe in a 1-2-3 cadence. This keeps a rhythm and steady pace. It also alternates which side is "1" which helps balance the force on each side of the body even if one leg is stronger than the other.

> Question 3: *Do my shoulders point straight to the ceiling?*
> Question 4: *Do I feel the same strength in my chest and upper back?*

Keep your rib cage lifted and chest forward. When you walk, lead with your chest to help the forward momentum of your body.

> Question 5: *Am I pulling my ribs in front down and lifting the ribs in back?*
> Question 6: *Is my chest more forward than my belly?*

Keep your abdominal muscles pulled in gently. By drawing in the abdominals as though you were pressing them towards the spine, you protect your lower back. If those muscles were slack, the pelvis would tip forward, the back would over-arch, and the muscles across your lower back would tighten and irritate your nerves. The abdominals also work as stabilizers and give additional strength to your body.

> Question 7: *Is my pubic bone pulling up and tail bone tilting down?*

Keep your knees soft. Do not lock the knee of your back leg as you walk. Roll all the way through your foot. Transfer the weight of your body from the heel through the middle part of your foot and into the toes.

> Question 8: *Are my leg muscles balanced so my knee is aligned and not stiff?*
> Question 9: *Are my feet balanced? Is the center of my body directly above my arches?*

Keep the body walking in a straight line. Put one foot directly in front of the other and find a comfortable stride, keeping your feet hip-width apart and moving towards the center line of your body. When you step out in front, be sure your knee does not extend forward of the middle of your foot. This ensures correct mechanics in your knee and powers you forward without any strain to the ligaments.

> Question 10: *Can I drop a plumb line from the ceiling and have it go down the center of each body segment in a straight line?*

To complete the technique, as your heel strikes the ground, it shifts from the outer part of your foot through the middle to the inside bottom part. This keeps your feet flexible enough to adjust to uneven terrain. Use your arms in a rhythmic, swinging motion. Arms should be positioned at about a 90-degree angle. Hands remain lightly closed. They should never swing up across your chest. Rely on your shoulders and hips to propel you forward, not your elbows and knees. The hips are relaxed and flexible. They shift back and forth.

Your Exercise Pulse Rate

As we age, our maximum attainable heart rate goes down. This means the capacity for our heart to work efficiently during aerobic activity goes down unless we do something about keeping it up. I'll show you how to find your fat-burning heart rate zone—the rate where your body burns calories most efficiently—and how to measure it during exercise.

I've always liked measurements. Showing an improvement is motivational. A daily aerobic workout is fun and you always feel better afterwards but it takes a lot of effort. I'll teach you the simplest way to take your own pulse to determine if you're working at the right pace and intensity that's within a safe range for your heart.

Being aerobically fit is a combination of how efficient our heart, lung and muscle capacity is in using oxygen and delivering it to the body to produce energy. We can measure the efficiency of our heart rate and be able to estimate the amount of calories we burn—our energy expenditure. It's satisfying to know you're burning all those extra calories.

When we take our pulse rate, we're measuring the regular beating in the arteries which is caused by the contractions of the heart. There are several tests you can easily take to monitor yourself before, during, and after the workout.

Resting Heart Rate
Measures cardiovascular fitness when you get out of bed in the morning. A low rate is desirable and you achieve this as your fitness increases. Depending on age and general health, a desirable rate is 60–75.

Recovery Heart Rate
Measure how much time it takes for your heart to slow down following a workout. You become more efficient and recover more quickly as your heart and lungs become conditioned.

Target Heart Rate
Measures the aerobic activity of your working body. Twenty minutes is the minimum time in this "training zone."

Maximum Heart Rate
Measures the fastest your heart can beat safely based on the theory that 220 is the maximum heart rate of a baby and that as we age this rate decreases by one beat per year. It is a factor in determining target heart rate but not the rate at which you should work out.

The formula, 220 minus your age, is not the rate at which you should work out. It's your maximum heart rate which you then multiply by a percentage between 60 and 80% to get your target heart rate.

A friend of mine who is twenty-five years younger than I am and a professional dancer introduced me to a new aerobic activity,

Use this Formula to Measure the Different Heart Rates

Use the fingertips of your second and third fingers to find either the carotid artery at the side of your neck, or the radial artery on the inside of your wrist. I can find the pulse in the neck easier than in the wrist.

1. Use a watch or clock with a sweep-second hand that is easy to see.
2. Place the two fingertips either at the side of your neck or at your wrist. You'll have to slide and press them gently around the area to pick up the pulse.

For the neck, turn your head side to side to feel the long strip of muscle (the sternocleido-mastoid) which runs from the sternum to the bone behind your ear. You'll find your pulse nestled in at the front of that muscle. I find it best using my right hand and turning my head slightly—about 30 degrees—to the left.

For the wrist, turn up your palm and press your fingertips on the inside of your wrist just below the wrist bone.

3. Take your pulse rate by counting the number of times your heart beats, which is a slight pulsing feeling at the pulse site. I like to take my pulse rate for ten seconds and multiply it by six because it's easy to measure ten seconds. But you can choose whichever counting method you like. Just be sure to have it as a ratio that equals sixty seconds, or one minute. Try out fifteen seconds times four beats; 6 seconds times 10 beats, etc.

spinning, where you simulate a strenuous bike ride while on a stationary bicycle. I have a high level of cardiovascular conditioning, but I wasn't paying attention to my heart rate and just followed my friend's pace and intensity. All of a sudden, I felt like my heart was bursting, a feeling I've never had during aerobic activities. I slowed down and took my pulse rate. It exceeded my maximum heart rate. If I had not been sensitive to how I was feeling, I could have damaged myself.

Simple Target Heart-Rate Chart

AGE	60%	70%	75%	80%
30	114	133	143	152
35	111	130	139	148
40	108	126	135	144
45	105	123	131	140
50	102	119	128	136
55	99	116	124	132
60	96	112	120	128
65	93	109	116	124
70	90	105	113	120
75	87	102	109	116
80	84	98	105	112
85	81	95	101	108
90	78	91	98	104

How to Determine Your Target Heart Rate

There are two distinct methods of measuring Target Heart Rate. One is shorter: 220 (MHR) minus age times workout intensity percentage (60%, 70%, 75% or 80%). For a forty year-old woman, that is 220 minus 40 equals 180 times 75% equals 135 beats per minute. See the Simple Target Heart-Rate Chart on this page.

I prefer the Karvonen formula. It is a little bit longer but is recommended by The American College of Sports Medicine. This method is more personalized, taking into account that each person's level of fitness is different. It calculates a percentage of the heart rate reserve: the difference between the resting heart rate and maximum heart rate.

THE KARVONEN FORMULA

Heart Rate Reserve equals Maximum HR minus Resting HR

You calculate your Target Heart Rate as a percentage of your Heart Rate Reserve, plus your Resting Heart Rate. You can see that by plugging in your personal resting Heart Rate, you're personalizing this measurement.

A 40 year old woman with a resting heart rate of 70, and age (approximate) related maximum heart rate of 220 - 40 = 180 (maximum HR), and an intensity level of 75% of maximum heart rate reserve would calculate her Target Heart Rate as follows:

180	(maximum heart rate)
- 70	
110	(heart rate reserve)
× .75	(% intensity)
82.5	
+ 70	(resting heart rate)
152.5	(target heart rate)

The Program

If you are new to walking, just go out for a walk and don't worry about your speed. Your goal is to work up to at least three miles in 30–60 minutes. Remember to keep your walking activity pleasurable so you'll stay with it.

To start, walk at least three times each week. When you're ready, make a daily walk part of your life. Even taking three walks of ten minutes each every day will get you to a beginning level.

Muscles need a few minutes to warm up and adapt to the task. Loosen every part of your body that you're going to use and get the circulation moving. Either roll and bend or use the Flexibility Program on page 83.

After you've finished your walk, you'll feel your muscles are warmed up. This might be an appropriate time to fit in your Stretch and Joint Looseners from Chapter Four.

Any long walk that you take for pleasure can be counted as your aerobic workout. But it must be sustained at a pace of 4 or 5 miles per hour, which is either a fifteen- or a twenty-minute mile. In the beginning, stay on the same course each time so you can measure your improvement. Walk slowly for the first few minutes and build up speed gradually. Shorter, quicker steps will increase your speed. In general, an easy to manage pace means you can walk longer and with this added time, burn more calories.

You're now ready to walk either three or four or five miles in approximately 15-minute miles. You'll get to know how each different pace feels. You can simply walk for time, feeling assured that you're covering an adequate distance.

- Start slowly to warm up and increase your speed after three minutes.
- Check that you're at the training rate after eight minutes.
- Continue for twenty to thirty minutes at that rate.
- Cool down for three minutes.
- Take your pulse rate as soon as you finish to check you were in the training zone.

FOUR-LEVEL WEEKLY WALKING SCHEDULE

Level	Distance	Time	Frequency
Level One	½–1 mile	any length of time	minimum 3 times
Level Two	1½–2 miles	30–40 minutes	minimum 5 times
Level Three	2–3 miles	40–60 minutes	every day
Level Four	3-plus miles	15 minute miles	every day

From time to time you may need to lessen the intensity, duration or frequency of your walk. Every activity that breaks a sedentary lifestyle is beneficial. You can walk a shorter distance, or a slower pace as long as you walk for 30 minutes. If you intend to walk every day and then miss a day or two a week, you'll still have five days of fitness.

Varying and Increasing Your Aerobics Workout

If you are a fitness beginner, start with a walking program. For more vigorous, higher-intensity activities, you have many choices.

The first is a combined walk and gentle jog workout. Alternate your pace spontaneously in order to vary your heart rate. This builds speed and endurance and promotes better recovery heart rate. Be sure you can carry on a conversation during the jog period.

The second is to choose a path that has some gentle hills to combine with the flatter surfaces. This has greater impact on your body than walking on flat surfaces alone. It increases your cardiovascular workload and offers natural resistance training. To increase your bone mass and bone density, it is recommended that you walk at an incline. Look for a route that offers some moderate hills. Begin with up to eight minutes on a flat surface, then stride up and down the hilly portions for twenty minutes and finish your walk on a more even surface. Explore the terrain available to you to make your walk as interesting and challenging as you can.

Adding extra weight to the body during exercise increases the intensity. But I don't recommend holding hand weights when you walk because this can cause tension in your neck and shoulders. The Muscle Memory Voice you use during your walk asks: "Is there a long space between my ear and shoulder?" Answer YES! No hunching and bunching, whatever you do.

However, to help you go beyond your present fitness level, you could try wearing a knapsack as your extra weight. Have you ever noticed how much harder your breathing is when you're carrying a heavy package up the stairs? This increase in cardiovascular output is something to work towards.

"Interval Training" is combining a higher intensity workout (at about 75–80% target heart rate) with a lower intensity workout (at about 60% target heart rate), for about five minutes each. Your heart rests during the lower intensity portion. With more vigorous, higher intensity activity, your metabolism is revved up, so you burn more calories.

Indoor Fitness

Plenty of opportunities exist for indoor aerobic fitness. Let's begin with skipping rope, a very strenuous activity that children used to do. It's something to do now when we're feeling hardy. You need an ordinary jump rope to start off with a basic skipping step. Believe me, this is strenuous and you have to be partial to skipping rope to keep up with this program. But some people like it, so if it sounds appealing (and challenging) give it a try!

Be sure to wear sneakers with good cushioning and support to protect your calves and shins against impact from the jumps. As you become more coordinated and accustomed to jumping, jump low to the ground.

I have a treadmill in my home which I enjoy very much. Treadmills—a moving belt on which you walk or jog—have become popular because they're easy to do at any level and are the most efficient indoor machines at maintaining your heart rate. There are a variety of treadmills which can be very sophisticated with lots of different computer programs: calorie expenditure calibrated and heart rate monitored. But the basic ability to measure your distance, time, and incline is enough to keep you interested.

At the beginning, use this suggested treadmill program. As your stamina and strength increase, you can vary your workout. Try alternating quicker and slower speeds and/or increase and decrease the incline—the height of your slope. When you decide on a challenging but comfortable speed and incline level, stay there for 10 minutes. Evaluate how you feel. Take your pulse rate, and check that it hasn't exceeded your target heart rate. Remember to stretch afterwards to prevent stiff muscles in your legs.

Work at a challenging rate, but keep your workout safe. While you are on your treadmill or whatever stationary equipment you can access, apply the Muscle Memory Quiz to get the most out of it.

Walking Works

I chose walking as the aerobic activity to recommend because it always feels comfortable to do and it's efficient. Some days you may notice your body feels stiffer than it used to and the thought of going for a jog doesn't sound great. But going out for a walk is natural and doesn't hurt. You can stay with a brisk 3-mile (4–5 miles an hour) walk or walk for 45 minutes on a hilly terrain.

The key word is STAY. What good is an exercise plan if you don't do it? To plan activity that sounds too stressful or too strenuous for you—like running or doing a machine that intimidates you—is counterproductive. In the time it takes to waver over the plans, you can get out and walk, be back, shower and be done.

At the beginning of my aerobic life, I just took the choice out of *whether* to do it or not. I left in the choice of *what* to do. Try this approach and see if it works for you. I think it will keep you

Skipping Rope

- Start week 1 with 5 minutes, 3 times a week. Be sure to check your pulse rate as you increase your time.
- By week 4, skip for 10 minutes 4 to 5 times a week.
- By week 8, skip for 15–20 minutes 5–6 times a week.

Treadmill Program

- The first two or three minutes are for your heart to adapt to the activity
- In eight minutes you're into your cardiovascular training zone. Stay in that zone for at least 20 minutes.
- The next 10-plus minutes you're in the fat burning zone.
- Then slow your pace to cool down to complete a 30–45 minute workout for a calorie expenditure of about 300 calories.

Walk Safely…

- Avoid slanting places so you can keep your body alignment even and not favor one side.
- Look for smooth surfaces. Be aware of where you place your foot to avoid injuries.
- In all weather, be sure to drink water before and after your walk. All your body systems function better when you drink the water you need.

involved and committed to a regular aerobic workout without any soreness or boredom.

The walking ritual becomes so personal that you'll recognize your different levels of exertion. The Borg Perceived Exertion Scale is sometimes used to measure and define your exertion level from very, very light to very, very hard. You will get to know your body's abilities very well on your own by paying attention to your pulse rate and how you feel. It's satisfying to become so finely tuned.

Now, I'd like your participation. I hope to bump into you on some country road or city street, an open beach or woodland trail and share an aerobic high!

…And Comfortably

- Choose the right walking shoes. Buy them at a store where employees can help you find the right shoe for your foot type. Don't go for a snug fit. There should be room to accommodate a space the width of your thumbnail between the toebox and the tip of your longest toe. I like shoes that are extra sturdy and stable with padding in the heel and the ball of the foot. They should be flexible and feel comfortable from the very beginning.
- Wear layered clothing so you can remove the top layer after you warm up. In colder weather, start off with gloves and a hat.

CHAPTER SEVEN

Mindsets and Exercises for Sensuality and Sexuality

Exercise, sensuality, and sexuality are all parts of feeling comfortable within your body. The exercises in this chapter target the muscles and joints you use for sensual opportunities. Think about increasing the intimacy between you and your body.

SENSUALITY FOREVER

To be a woman is to be sensuous. Sensuality is about pleasuring your body, not only with sex, but through many areas of your life. Anything that enhances the senses is sensual. Sensual and creative energy can be deeply experienced in your work, companions, relationships, free time and private time. Feeling good, vital and pleased with yourself—satisfying your appetites—leads to gratification and pleasure.

Women are nurturers. Learn to nurture yourself. Take the time to relax and beautify your body. Each body has its own erogenous zones. Discover which of your zones make you feel good. You can do self-massage, exchange massage with a partner or hire a massage therapist to touch and release feelings in your body.

Keep your skin soft and nice to feel. Skin is very susceptible to touch. Stimulating it by touch increases circulation and body heat, both of which feel good. Warm baths or showers keep your skin hydrated and are relaxing to your entire body. If the sense of smell is pleasing to you, use scented bath salts or bubbles to heighten your enjoyment. And if time for relaxation is short, maximize it. Rather than a bath or shower, moisten a cloth or sponge and freshen yourself. Then lie down with your feet up and spend a few quiet moments breathing and floating. Either wear a comfortable robe or shirt or a bra and panties. You might even enjoy lying naked enjoying the contours of your body.

You can create a feeling similar to being pampered in a spa. Surround yourself with pleasing objects, especially wherever you spend a lot of time. Perk up your bedroom and bath with some new things to beautify those environments. Check that the lighting is pleasing to you. Three fourths of the world—and three fourths of your body—is water. Keep crystal clear water nearby. It can be a natural aphrodisiac.

Your Five Senses

Sensuality is the experience of getting in touch with the five senses. Invoke and bring them into your life often. Vary the stimuli around you. Eyes are powerful receptors. Be deliberate and see everything. Notice what's new as you reaquaint yourself with familiar sights.

Touch and feel the way your body moves and stay connected with it. Wear clothing that feels good against your skin. The nerve endings in your fingertips make them very sensitive. Take advantage of this.

Be aware of how the environment affects you. Sometimes you've probably noticed "there's a feeling in the air." Recall a gentle, warm breeze or the tingling of a crisp autumn day. Nature's light, changing through the day and the seasons, elicits different moods and feelings.

Smell, one of the strongest senses that reawakens lots of memories, increases pleasure in many ways. Introduce provocative scents into your life either with flowers, aromatic oils and candles or an aromatherapy massage.

Hear beautiful music, listen to the sounds around you or simply enjoy the lovely silence. That same breeze which feels good also sounds delightful. When beats of music permeate and enliven your body, the sensual experience is enhanced.

Eat something that satisfies your appetite not only nutritionally, but sensually. A ripe peach, eaten slowly, just like they do in all those French films, can be very sensual. Savor the textures, intense flavors and enticing smells of all the special foods you eat.

What Makes You Feel Good?

Think of even more ways to arouse your senses. Perpetuate the quality of your life by satisfying your innermost desires.

A student told me that one day when she was harried and frustrated in her office, she skipped lunch and went to the beauty parlor. She came out feeling wonderful. A nice lunch and a short walk would be just as soothing. Do whatever you can to pull yourself out of a low mood. It's great to be able to do something for yourself.

While I work out, I like to wear a body lotion that smells so fresh and clean it inspires my physicality. Ask yourself what you might bring to your workout to make it more physical and sensual. Let your workout by your private love affair with yourself.

I want you to feel like the strong, wise, sexy woman you are. Eleanora Lipton, R.P.P., Director, Atlanta Polarity Center, agrees. She and I have conducted spa weeks together where we've witnessed the inspiring effects this meditation has on women from all walks of life.

ELEANORA'S SENSUAL MEDITATION

Meditation has many levels, shapes and forms. The first step is visualization. We are always visualizing something. In meditation, however, we choose a focus that will create a desired feeling.

Find a comfortable, quiet place to lie down. Take a deep breath and scan your body to make sure that every part of you feels physically relaxed. Take another deep breath. As you relax more and more, your position will naturally shift. Allow your body to move just as it wishes.

As you breathe, imagine that you're in the most beautiful place in nature. This may or may not be somewhere you have experienced. You may notice that you begin to feel more relaxed.

Breathe the air and feel the qualities of this most beautiful place. Take another deep breath and look deeper into this landscape.

Explore the leaves of the trees, the petals of the flowers, the waves of the ocean or the crevices of the mountains. Feel the sand in your toes or a warm breeze on your skin.

Let your senses delight. Let your breath flow. And let your body relax even more.

Now imagine that with every inhalation, the qualities of your landscape are like a fine mist showering your whole body. With every exhalation, this energy feeds into every cell of your being—loving, nurturing and embracing you.

Bathe in this energy as long as you can. If you have a time limit, set an alarm so your mind is free.

Be with yourself every day and you will discover how much more you have to share and how much more connected you feel with yourself. This is the key to being a sensual beautiful woman.

SEXUAL ENERGY

Whether for sensual thoughts or sexual activities, focus on the woman inside of you. You don't have to engage in the sexual act to feel sexy. Sexuality is a byproduct of your emotions and state of mind. Why give up thinking about intimacy? Intimate thoughts and actions stimulate chemical reactions that propel the body into heightened awareness and enjoyment. Visualize pleasurable moments that will stimulate chemical activity in your brain.

When you shower, fix your hair and check your general appearance, you like to feel and look good. It's nice to hear compliments. What's your image? How do you choose to present yourself? Creative? Athletic? Sensitive? Intelligent? Feminine, attractive ... sexy? Maybe all of the above. It's interesting and mysterious to change the way you look.

Femininity can add excitement to your life. One female lawyer in the studio has to dress very conservatively and plainly for work. Because this image goes against her nature, she's figured out that wearing very sexy underwear makes her feel more like herself. Experiment with the lingerie you wear. Discover what puts you in the mood and increases your sex appeal.

Ongoing Sexuality

It's nice to move in a way that activates our sexual energy. There's a dancing club across the street from where I live. In spite of the fact that the club does not serve any liquor, wine or beer, I see people leaving there when I look out my window at 7 A.M. Dancing can feel as stimulating as the sex act.

Wake up and unwrap your sexuality. If we give up thinking about sex, we can lose muscle awareness in parts of our body. Being sexually aroused, whether alone or with a partner, may help maintain vaginal health because of the lubrication and elasticity of the vagina. Sexual contact and intimacy help us feel younger. Studies are under way looking into the sexuality of older women. For the first time, the research establishment seems to recognize that older women are sexual. Although previous studies have usually focused on young woman, there are many women enjoying sex at every age.

Exercise and Sex

It's likely you'll have increased energy from the Daily Ten work-out. If you like, you can translate this into increased sexual appetite. A conditioned body has more stamina for sex. There's a "feedback" mechanism between being sexual and being fit. Feeling strong and healthy is sexy and being sexual makes you want to be fit and toned. Strength and flexibility enable you to participate with more ease. For example, doing the Positive Push-Ups in the Daily Ten will give you the arm strength to be on top more easily. You'll be able to enjoy a variety of sexual positions when you are stronger and more flexible. And, having better cardiovascular conditioning gives you more endurance for all activities.

Try to transmit sexual energy throughout your body. Rhythmic movements have an arousing and tranquilizing effect on you. Contracting the several sets of muscles inside along the pelvic floor gives you a pleasurable feeling of tightness in your vagina. Tense and relax your vaginal muscles and think of that sexual energy traveling up through your spine. Pump your buttocks to increase sexual feelings. Moving your pelvis and hips awakens your sensuality.

Feeling Comfortable

Most women love romance. Many of us like to read about sensuality and sexuality and want to experience it in our own lives. Sexual thoughts or fantasies are one way to get in the mood.

Sexual communication begins long before bodies are undressed. Do whatever makes you comfortable in new situations. You don't have to disrobe until you're ready.

Some sexual positions are more comfortable and enjoyable than others, especially if you have back pain or other injuries. Work together with your partner and experiment to see what feels pleasurable. Try to be in a position which supports your back. You can lie on your back and raise your knees as your partner uses hands, arms, or knees for support and to prevent putting too much weight on you. Lying on your sides with knees bent or having sex on all fours may be comfortable. Use pillows for support and stability.

The P.C. Muscle

At least three of the Daily Ten exercises target the abdominals. It's extremely important to keep these muscles strong, both for appearance and function. The lower abdominals, several ligaments, tendons and the muscles deep within the pelvic floor help support the internal organs. One pelvic floor muscle, the pubococcygeal—P.C. Muscle—supports the pelvis. It also contracts during arousal and sexual orgasm. The P.C. goes between the pubic bone and tailbone. With exercise, you'll notice an improvement in muscle tone in this area. You can even use commercial products that act like weights, whereby squeezing the P.C., you prevent the weight from dropping. The P.C. Tightener in this chapter accomplishes the same strengthening.

Your Breasts

Aesthetic and therapeutic concepts combine again. We touch our breasts for self-examinations to augment our yearly breast exams. Notice how smooth your breasts feel when you touch them.

There are changes in the breast tissue as we get older. Exercise will help keep the breasts lifted. Strong chest muscles support the breasts in the same way as a good uplift bra. It makes sense that strengthening all the muscles around the breasts can help hold them up regardless of changes in the tissue. When your shoulders and upper back are straight from your exercise commitment, there's additional support.

The Shoulder Circles and Positive Push-Ups in your Daily Ten will not only strengthen your pectorals, they will also improve the look of your breasts. Think of using your chest muscles in a motion similar to tightening a bra strap. Even women who have had breast surgery tell me these exercises make them feel balanced.

THE PROGRAM

The genital muscles are private, delicate and can be exercised to get stronger. When you improve the muscle tone around the vagina, you can be muscle specific when you want that feeling. Choose an intimate environment as you exercise your pelvis, with the intent of heightening your sensuality. Use the breathing techniques you've learned to relax and enjoy your body.

Through these three exercises, bring Muscle Memory with you, target the pelvic muscles and enjoy!

The P.C. Tightener

When you improve the muscle tone around the vagina,
you have much better control of that area. Move your hands from
the cord-like tendon between the upper thigh and pubic
bone on to your lower belly. Enjoy the connection as you contract
the pelvic floor muscles. Instruction #4 isolates the P.C.
(pubococcygeal) for specific strengthening.
Do this exercise lying on your back and then face down to learn
to isolate the different muscles. To heighten your sensuality,
keep the motions slow and rhythmic. Then do the P.C. Tightener
while standing and feel yourself counteracting the force of
gravity by lifting from your inside.

Note: This may seem similar to the Kegel exercise done during pregnancy. However the P.C. Tightener aims for additional sexual pleasure.

On Back:

Position
Lie on your back, knees bent, feet on floor hip-width apart.

Instructions
1. Begin by tensing the upper thigh-pubic tendon and use its connection into the pubic bone to pull in all your lower abdominals.
2. Place hands on lower belly and feel hips pull together as you contract the transverse muscle across the waist. (Figure 1)
3. Breath naturally and hold for a slow count of five. Release smoothly and repeat five times.
4. Relax abdominals and concentrate on the vaginal area. Squeeze in at the pelvic opening to isolate the P.C., which feels like tightening around a man's penis or a finger inserted into you. Hold for three seconds and repeat 10 times.

   As you gain greater control of the P.C., squeeze the P.C. for 10 seconds and repeat three times.
5. Drop one leg down at time and turn over onto your belly.

On Belly:

Position
Lie on your belly. Rest forehead on hands.

Instructions
1. Squeeze buttocks muscles together and push down to press pubic bone into floor.
2. Draw in the transverse muscle and upper thigh-pubic tendon and lift your waist slightly off floor. (Figure 2)
3. Feel a pleasurable tightening of your vaginal area and hold for a slow count of five. Release, then repeat five to ten times.
4. Raise up to hands and knees. Round over and sit back on heels to relax the lower back and prepare for the next exercise.

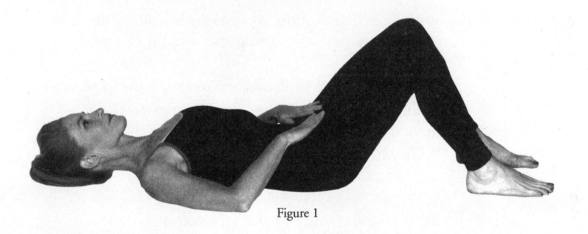

Figure 1

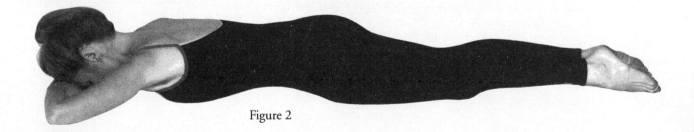

Figure 2

Butt Swirls

Working your pelvis and hip area awakens your sensuality. This delicate, private part of you needs attention in a feminine way. As you increase your flexibility, you'll feel more comfortable in a variety of positions. Rather than using your muscles to move your bones, as you do throughout the rest of the Muscle Memory Method, use your bones as the primary movers. Let your pubic bone, hip bones and tailbone control and swirl your pelvis as fluidly as a well-trained belly dancer.

Position

Stand with your legs about two feet apart, knees slightly bent and toes turned slightly out. Imagine a small hoola hoop around your hips and don't let it drop towards your ankles.

Instructions

1. Place hands on hips and press pubic bone to touch front of hoop.

2. With a circling motion, move right hip along the rim of the imaginary hoop and pause when it's by your side. (Figure 1)

3. Now, slowly swirl your tailbone to touch the back rim.

4. Leading with your left hip, continue the motion. (Figure 2)

5. Pause when the left hip is by your side and then complete the swirl. Repeat three times and then swirl in the opposite direction.

6. Bring your feet together and rock your pelvis forward and back to relax your muscles and complete your workout.

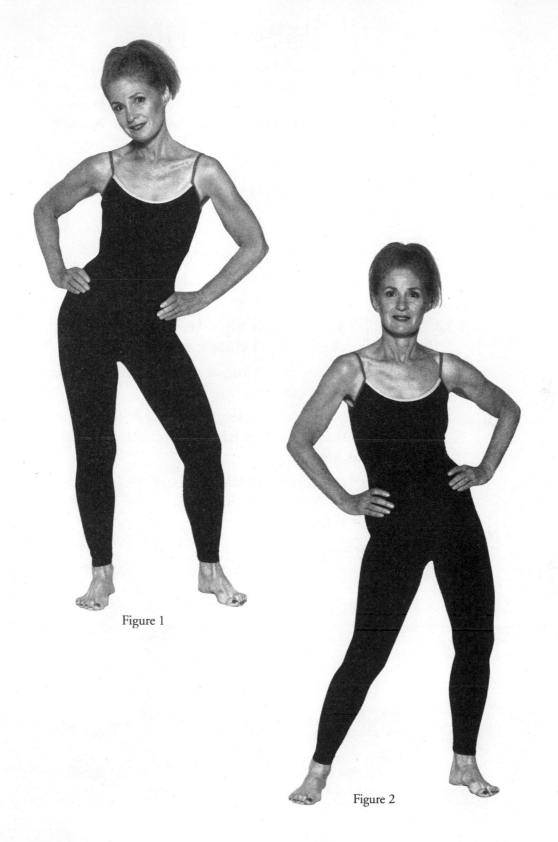

Figure 1

Figure 2

Tailbone Tilt

Lifting the tailbone high puts your pelvis in a position
that increases circulation in your genital area. Although sexual activity
is not considered an exercise, it does require oxygen and energy.
Lifting the tailbone feels great under any circumstances because it
stretches out your lower back muscles.

Note: Immediately after the birth of a child, substitute additional P.C. Tighteners for the Tailbone Tilt. The inverted position of the Tailbone Tilt allows air to get sucked in. This is a pleasurable feeling. But it is dangerous for postpartum women until the uterus shrinks and goes back into the pelvis. Please check with your doctor.

Position
With knees on floor, round body over and sit back
on your heels.

Instructions
1. Open knees wide apart and stretch arms diagonally forward to the "11" and "1" on the face of a clock. Forehead and fingertips down on floor.

2. As you lift your tailbone high, keep it behind knees and slide your arms and chest forward on a slant.

3. Turn head to one side, sink in between your shoulder blades and rest chest on floor. (Figure 1)

4. Slowly sway hips from side to side in a rocking motion to feel the flexibility in pelvic floor muscles. Pause as each hip is lifted high.

5. Repeat several times and then sit back on heels and round over. Keep your abdominals pulled in and feel your back stretch.

6. Either Squat to Stand or Tuck to Stand.

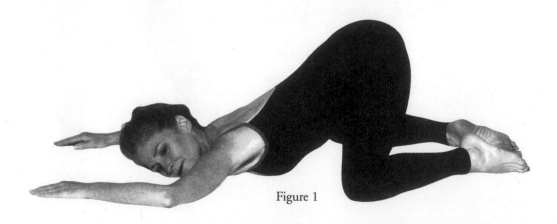

Figure 1

The Self-Directed Woman

The Self-Directed Woman

I encourage you to make the effort to discover who you are and what's important in your life. A student of mine said, "I am the cake and everything else in my life is the icing." Take the time to strengthen your identity. Enlarge your ambitions and open up your sense of wonder and creativity.

You came to this book interested in making a fitness commitment and I hope I have made it easier and more enjoyable for you. Exercise will help you keep a healthy lifestyle. Perhaps the changes in your fitness can inspire you toward other important changes you'd like to make. Knowledge about your body can lead to self-discovery and new perceptions.

Now that you've learned the magic of Muscle Memory, the method is yours forever. You've developed the skills to be gentle with your body but firm when you tell your muscles what to do. Apply these skills to whatever new interests you choose.

Your ways of living affect not only how healthy, but also how happy you are. Exercise is a way to reduce tension and free up energy, making your body more active and rejuvenating your mind. Emotional issues can sap your energy. Nurturing the body and soul strengthens your emotional foundation.

Keeping It Going

If in the past you've had trouble keeping a program going, this time will be different. Your mind is involved and the results you see will keep you motivated. What fitness level would please you for the rest of your life?

Fitness is not an obsession for me but it is a passion and I'm able to make the time for it. Exercise can fit into anyone's life without taking it over. But if you have occasional difficulty fitting exercise in, don't let it become a burden. I tell my students, *"take the choice out."* It's much better to do even a little every day for your health than to do nothing. Even the most committed-to-exercise people fall off track sometimes but they get back on faster.

Having a good body is not a gift bestowed on a lucky few. It results from a commitment towards fitness and health. Use the wisdom and intelligence of your mind and body in the Muscle Memory program to keep it going.

Staying Healthy

A combination of ongoing exercise, healthy nutrition, stress reduction, and adequate rest will lead to wellness and vitality. These are the most practical ways to avoid common health problems. Taking responsibility for your own health is the best health care plan you can have.

Acknowledge the synergy between exercise and diet. Plan a routine and aim for balance in both. Your body loves balance. Vary your muscle groups and your food groups every day. You know what habits are unhealthy and you know you can change them. Healthier habits can keep you physiologically younger.

A good night's sleep feels great. Deep sleep gives body systems a rest and cells a chance to restore themselves. The Three Minute Breathing Relaxation can help quiet your mind to prepare for sleep. Aerobic exercise that uses up a lot of energy during the day also contributes to restful slumber. A warm bath raises your body temperature and can make you sleepy. And slipping in a half-hour nap every now and then can be very refreshing.

Sometimes travel compromises our health. It can be difficult to find healthy food or the time to work out. Your sleep patterns can be disturbed. You may feel people or circumstances are thwarting your efforts. Don't become frustrated; be flexible. Drink lots of water throughout the day. Try to use walking as your mode of transportation. Connect with your Muscle Memory Voice wherever you are. And the Daily Ten, or a portion of it, can fit into just about any room.

Growing Better

You're at the pivotal age where you can create a blueprint for your older years. Things change in your mind's eye. Try to create your own perspective on the changes in your body and attitudes. Age is a perception, defined in part by the degree of health and well being you feel. Muscle tone and mental tuning come from having an active life. Make a plan to keep going.

Some natural gifts diminish with age, but others blossom as you get older. Now you can make yourself the focus of your care. And with the Muscle Memory Method, you'll have more strength and stamina to take care of all your other responsibilities.

You can accomplish what you want when you visualize it and allow yourself to overcome any past obstacles. Put a different spin on the problem and reconstruct your approach to it. There's always enough time to take another stab at a cherished goal. Changes and new challenges can be hard but most often they're worth it.

Physical, mental, emotional, and spiritual changes occur all the time. Our paths shift and evolve. Keep focused on your most important issues and, please, be patient and kind to yourself. Take the time to figure out what your deepest psychological being is. Acknowledge you have a separate life from other people.

Embracing a New Decade

Prior to celebrating my 50th birthday, I indulged in a fantasy about an exotic vacation or a sensational party. But after several months of indecision, I chose a four-day hiking trip. I've always felt healthy, real, and alive while in the mountains. After a wonderfully physical and aesthetic time, I realized that I'd have more satisfaction in my life if I could fit hiking into my schedule.

Think about what you like to do for pleasure. Maybe because I've played piano all my life, I love to listen to music. Now when I do my aerobic workout listening to Mick Jagger singing, "You can't always get what you want but if you try, you get what you need," the message is clear and inspirational. Visualize how you want to look and feel at this point in your life. Bannish any thoughs that say you can't look good as you get older. Applaud your efforts.

Now we know we can achieve our goals. It's vital to decide what they are and to take time to rethink them. As I grew up, my dad often quoted Somerset Maugham. "It's a funny thing about life. If you refuse to accept anything but the best, you very often get it."

Managing Time

Try to make enough time to do all the things that you want. My friend and colleague Jane Cooper, M.S.W., shared her Time-Managing Technique with my students. Try it for yourself now.

Jane tells us, "We generally feel content when we spend time on the things that are important to us. When we spend time on things that aren't meaningful, we feel dissatisfied."

Apart from work and sleep, you have 35 percent of your time left, or 8.4 hours every day. Surprised? Sure, you have to commute, eat, and take care of many responsibilities. But with 8.4 hours you can do those things and more.

Self-Imaging

Appreciate your body each morning when you arise, regardless of your mood. Visualize the natural beauty and shape of your muscles. Give energy back to your body. Be grateful and thank it for the day to come.

Jane's Time-Managing Technique

1. List the five things in your life that are most important. For example, health, family, financial security, etc.
2. Figure out how you spend your time. One day, 24 hours, equals 100 percent. For example, work is 35 percent or 8.4 hours. Sleep takes 30 percent or 7.2 hours. You have 35 percent left.
3. Compare the data and you'll be able to see how your life matches your values.
4. If there's a discrepancy, maybe it's time to reassess how you spend your time and make some decisions.

I've always lived a healthy lifestyle. But sometimes my jeans get too tight and I feel frustrated. At those times, I rely on the kind relationship I've developed with my body. One thing I might do is take a hot shower and massage myself with body lotion afterwards. Then, rather than looking unhappily into the mirror, I do the Muscle Memory Boost and feel the connection into my center, knowing it's intact. Be confident that you can look good at any size because the Muscle Memory Method keeps you aligned and lovely.

In Chapter Seven, I suggested you relax being naked and enjoy the contours of your body. There are times when you may feel there's nothing to enjoy! But try to look at your best features because that's what other people usually see first. You'll feel much better when you learn to appreciate yourself. Accept compliments graciously and never put yourself down.

We all know there really is something to "positive thinking." A sense of humor and an optimistic attitude—as often as possible—can serve you well. Measure your success by how you've grown into the woman you are now. Respect your accomplishments and add them to your life skills. Never underestimate yourself. We gain life experience and hope to gain wisdom as we age.

Memories

As we reflect on our past experiences, it's the happy memories that sustain us. Even painful memories about a loved one who died, a relationship you lost or a satisfying career that ended can subside when you're ready to substitute more pleasant memories of them.

Childhood memories are as varied as we are. Having little experience dealing with pain as a youngster, I was surprised and unprepared for the ups and downs I had no control over as an adult. After being tempted to cope through illusion and fantasy, I stayed centered through just the sort of physical, spiritual, and intellectual regimen I've recommended to you: the Muscle Memory Method.

Memories from events that are important enough to be remembered are part of each of our histories. Jane Cooper has an excellent technique to help you recall positive history in your own life and use it to succeed in the present.

Re-Programming the Mind

Taking the Muscle Memory Quiz and learning to use the Muscle Memory Voice to re-program your muscles is like a guided meditation.

Jane's Library Technique

By the time we reach adulthood, we all have a kind of personal tape library in our minds about who we are. We keep replaying those tapes all through our lives.

Some of them help us to set and achieve goals, but others lower self-esteem and destroy confidence.

Take the time to review these "re-runs" and decide which to keep and which to "re-shoot."

It's a mistake to let old, outdated roles prevent you from present and future success and happiness.

You've taught both your mind and your muscles to remember. You'll remember what's useful to you each day. You've retrained your mind to think in different ways and your muscles to work differently.

In the past, the brain was thought of as a machine. Conventional thinking said there was not much you could do to keep the brain active and alert as you aged. But that thinking is changing. Continued exposure to the same information increases our ability to remember. It's been shown that the number of connections in the brain can grow if you use your mind every day and continue the learning process. Exercise makes a strong contribution to this, too.

You've demonstrated this to yourself by learning the new language of Muscle Memory. It will not only keep you looking good, it will keep your mind sharp and involved.

The Beginning

We've come to the end of the book. But this is the beginning of the Muscle Memory Method for you.

Can you imagine how I feel when a forty-five year old woman comes into the studio and asks me if it's too late for her to benefit from exercise? Perhaps not, because you don't know that I have a few ninety-year-old students, many in their eighties, seventies and sixties and a younger contingent, too. I've seen exercise make a world of difference to all of them and I know it can do the same for you.

Consider the ways physicality can add pizzazz and enthusiasm to your life. Each of us can find herself on the verge of a re-awakening.

We have a desire to control our own lives. Creativity and authority are within each of us. With strong and healthy bodies, our potential is expanded. Be clear and honest about what's important. Feel comfortable striving towards those ends. Put a high stamp of approval on yourself and value who you are.

One last thought and that is to thank you for trying the Muscle Memory Method. It's been a magical time for me to share my lifelong work with you. Congratulations on your efforts. I assure you that you now have the tools for a strong, firm, younger body.

Acknowledgments

The Authors

Our agent, Susan Zeckendorf, deserves more thanks than could fit in an entire book.

We're grateful to Betty Anne Crawford, our editor, for her superior knowledge and humor.

We heartily thank our publisher, George de Kay, our publicist Darcie Rowan, production manager Rik Lain, and all the great people at M. Evans and Company.

Enormous thanks go to George Kerrigan for his outstanding cover and interior photography and to Roman Szolkowski for his terrific illustrations. We also thank Gayle Miller of Capezio for dressing Marjorie Jaffe, and Abigail Booth for hair and make-up magic. Thanks to Annemarie Redmond for her stylish book design and to Paul Perlow for his catchy cover. And to Hudson Copy and Duplications for their sharp work on short notice.

For assistance and support we could not have done without, our deepest appreciation to: Marilyn J. Abraham; Wendy Bass; Mary Ann Eckels; James R. Harris; Kathleen Kelly-Mazza; Laurie Kraman; Paula Dolata; Chris Martinez; Emil Micha; Madge Rosenberg; Dominick A. Sgammato; Mary P. Sgammato; Pamela Dean Strickler; and Bobbi, Jerry, and David Sherman.

We're appreciative of Anna Salo, M.S.P.T., for her careful review of our book.

We'd like to thank our respective attorneys, Steve Rand and Jerome J. Cohen.

Marjorie Jaffe

I am deeply grateful for the opportunity to work with Jo Sgammato. I feel as though God sent an angel to help me write a book that comes from my heart, my brain, and my memories.

A special thanks to Dr. Sonya Weber, my mentor, who always taught me that exercise works.

I am blessed with a supportive and loving family who share my passion for fitness, health, and joy: my husband, Jerry; children, Ian and Bryce; Mom, Rena; Uncle Mac; Mother-in-law, Terry; and my brother Ken and his family.

I've had the good fortune of working alongside many wonderful experts in the health and fitness fields. I am grateful to Jane Cooper, Edwige Gilbert, and Eleanora Lipton, who have contributed to this book, and to Mary Leck, who enriched my breathing and relaxation. Thanks to the teachers at Back in Shape and Spa Week colleagues for your inspiration and professional and moral support.

Thanks to Dr. Sharon Lewin who always took the time away from her busy practice to answer questions and support The Muscle Memory Method. And to Janice Hopkins Tanne, whose fax and telephone machines spoke with mine regularly about the most recent and cutting-edge medical news. And to Dr. Carol Livoti for her wise advice.

A special thanks to my brilliant and stylish close friends who were always willing to help. And the marvelously intelligent Back in Shape community who helped me make sure that each and every exercise would be satisfying and easy to follow. To the Tuesday and Thursday "10:30s," many of whom have been following the method for 20 years, thanks for your vision and experience and enthusiastic reaction to the Sensuality and Sexuality chapter!

Sincere thanks to Jacques d'Amboise who responds enthusiastically whenever asked for his support. And to U.S. Congresswoman Carolyn Maloney and the other busy women who have endorsed our program.

Thank you to Nick Dejnega, owner, and the staff at the Regency Spa in Hallandale, Florida, for rejuvenation, good food and rest, and to Dr. Frank Sabatino for his expertise and stimulating lectures.

Thank you, Shari James, for helping during every phase of this book.

Jo Sgammato

Marjorie Jaffe is the first and only exercise teacher to make me love exercise. She is a real pro and one terrific woman. Writing this book was a wonderful experience in commitment, friendship, and fun.

Special thanks to Ann Daly, who gave me the brochure that led me to Marjorie Jaffe's studio back in 1991. My neck and shoulders are especially grateful.

To my husband, Ira Fraitag, thanks for showing me that taking risks pays off.

My parents, Mary A. and Dominick A. Sgammato, my sister Mary P. Sgammato, and all the members of my family deserve my love and gratitude.

Thanks to Karla Dougherty for showing the true class that money can't buy.

My dear friends and professional colleagues helped with this book in immeasurable ways. Thanks pals!

Every Exercise—and Where to Find It

Index